Obsessive Compulsive Disorder

The latest assessment and treatment strategies

Third Edition

Gail Steketee, Ph.D.

Teresa Pigott, M.D.

Todd Schemmel, Ph.D., Contributing Author

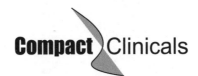

This book is intended for use by properly trained and licensed mental health professionals, who already possess a solid education in psychological theory, research, and treatment. This book is in no way intended to replace or supplement such training and education, nor is it to be used as the sole basis for any decision regarding treatment. It is merely intended to be used by such trained and educated professionals as a review and resource guide when considering how to best treat patients with obsessive compulsive disorder.

Obsessive Compulsive Disorder

The latest assessment and treatment strategies

Third Edition

by

Gail Steketee, Ph.D., and Teresa Pigott, M.D.

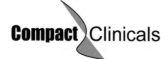

Published by: Compact Clinicals
                7205 NW Waukomis Dr., Suite A
                Kansas City, MO 64151
                816-587-0044

©2006 Dean Psych Press Corp. d/b/a Compact Clinicals

Prior releases: ©1999, 2003 by Gail Steketee, Ph.D., Teresa A. Pigott, M.D., and Todd Schemmel, Ph.D. cand.

Medical Editing: Kathi Whitman, In Credible English, Inc.,® Kansas City, Missouri

Book Design: Coleridge Design, Kansas City, Missouri

Library of Congress Cataloging in Publication data:

Steketee, Gail
Obsessive compulsive disorder : the latest assessment and treatment strategies / by Gail Steketee, Teresa A. Pigott.
        p.   ;   cm.
    Includes bibliographical references and index.
    ISBN-13: 978-1-887537-28-5
    ISBN-10: 1-887537-28-7
    1. Obsessive-compulsive disorder. I. Pigott, Teresa A., 1958-
II. Title.

    RC533.O2732 2006
    618.85'227–dc22
            2005037534

10 9 8 7 6 5 4 3 2 1

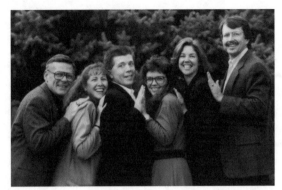

Our "Compacted" Compact Clinicals Team

Dear Valued Customer,

WELCOME to Compact Clinicals. We are committed to bringing mental health professionals up-to-date diagnostic and treatment information in a compact, timesaving, and easy-to-read format. Our line of books provides current, thorough reviews of assessment and treatment strategies for mental disorders.

We've "compacted" complete information for diagnosing each disorder and comparing how different theoretical orientations approach treatment. Our books use nonacademic language, real-world examples, and well-defined terminology.

Enjoy this and other timesaving books from Compact Clinicals.

Sincerely,

Melanie Dean, Ph.D.
President

Compact Clinicals Line of Books

Compact Clinicals currently offers these condensed reviews for professionals:

For Clinicians

Attention Deficit Hyperactivity Disorder
The latest assessment and treatment strategies

C. Keith Conners, Ph.D.

Bipolar Disorder
The latest assessment and treatment strategies

Trisha Suppes M.D., Ph.D., and Ellen B. Dennehy, Ph.D.

Borderline Personality Disorder
The latest assessment and treatment strategies

Melanie Dean, Ph.D.

Conduct Disorders
The latest assessment and treatment strategies

J. Mark Eddy, Ph.D.

Depression in Adults
The latest assessment and treatment strategies

Anton Tolman, Ph.D.

Obsessive Compulsive Disorder
The latest assessment and treatment strategies

Gail Steketee, Ph.D., and Teresa Pigott, M.D.

Post-Traumatic and Acute Stress Disorders
The latest assessment and treatment strategies

Matthew Friedman, M.D., Ph.D.

For Physicians

Bipolar Disorder: Treatment and Management
Trisha Suppes, M.D., Ph.D., and Paul E. Keck, Jr., M.D.

Read Me First

As a mental health professional, often the information you need can only be obtained after countless hours of reading or library research. If your schedule precludes this time commitment, Compact Clinicals is the answer.

Our books are practitioner oriented with easy-to-read treatment descriptions and examples. Compact Clinicals books are written in a nonacademic style. Our books are formatted to make the first reading, as well as ongoing reference, quick and easy. You will find:

▶ **Anecdotes** — Each chapter contains a fictionalized account that personalizes the disorder entitled, "From the Patient's Perspective."

▶ **Sidebars** — Narrow columns on the outside of each page highlight important information, preview upcoming sections or concepts, and define terms used in the text.

▶ **Definitions** — Terms are defined in the sidebars where they originally appear in the text and in an alphabetical glossary on pages 77 through 82.

▶ **References** — Numbered references appear in the text following information from that source. Full references appear on pages 83 through 95.

▶ **Case Examples** — Our examples illustrate typical adult client comments or conversational exchanges that help clarify different treatment approaches. Identifying information in the examples (e.g., the individual's real name, profession, age, and/or location) has been changed to protect the confidentiality of those clients discussed in case examples.

▶ **Key Concepts** — At the end of each chapter, we include a review list of key concepts from that chapter. Use these lists for ongoing quick reference as well as for reviewing what you learned from reading the chapter.

Contents

Chapter One:

Overview of Obsessive Compulsive Disorder   **I**

   How Common is OCD? 2

   What is the Likelihood of Recovery? 4

Chapter Two:

Diagnosing Obsessive Compulsive Disorder   **7**

   What Criteria are Used to Diagnose Obsessive Compulsive Disorder (OCD)? . . .7

   What are the Typical Characteristics of Those with OCD? 9

   What Tools are Available for Clinical Assessment? 10

      Clinical Interviews 10

         Medical History 10

         Individual and Family Psychiatric History 11

         Social and Occupational Functioning 12

         Role of Relatives 12

         Patient Insight 13

      Self-Report Instruments and Structured Interviews 13

      Behavior Assessment 14

      Psychometric Assessments 15

      Laboratory/Physical Exam Findings 15

   What Differentiates OCD from Other Disorders? 15

      Addictive Disorders 16

      Anxiety Disorder Due to a General Medical Condition 16

      Body Dysmorphic Disorder 16

      Delusional Disorder or Psychotic Disorder Not Otherwise Specified 17

      Generalized Anxiety Disorder, Panic Disorder, or Post-Traumatic Stress Disorder . . .17

      Hypochondriasis 17

      Major Depressive Episode 18

      Obsessive Compulsive Personality Disorder 18

      Phobias 18

      Schizophrenia 19

      Substance-Induced Anxiety Disorder 19

      Superstitions and Repetitive Checking Behaviors 19

      Tics 19

Chapter Three:

Psychosocial Treatments for Obsessive Compulsive Disorder   21

What Social and Psychological Influences May Cause OCD? 22

What is the Behavior Therapy Approach to Treating OCD? 23

   Behavioral Treatment Methods 23

      Early Behavioral Treatments 24

      Exposure and Response Prevention. 26

   Efficacy of Behavioral Treatment Approaches 29

      Initial OCD Behavioral Treatments 29

      Exposure and Response Prevention 30

What is the Cognitive Therapy Approach to Treating OCD? 32

   Cognitive Treatment Methods 33

      Rational Emotive Therapy (RET) 34

      Beck's Cognitive Therapy 35

   Efficacy of Cognitive Treatment Approaches 36

What is the Psychoanalytic Approach to Treating OCD? 37

   Psychoanalytic Treatment Methods 38

   Efficacy of Psychoanalytic Treatment Approaches .39

What is the Group Therapy Approach to Treating OCD? 39

   Group Therapy Treatment Methods 40

      Psychoeducational Group Therapy 41

      Behavioral Treatment Group Therapy 43

   Efficacy of Group Therapy 45

What is the Family Therapy Approach to Treating OCD? 46

   Family Therapy Treatment Methods 46

   Efficacy of Family Therapy Approaches 48

Chapter 4:

Medical Treatment for Obsessive Compulsive Disorder   51

What is the Role of Genetics in the Development of OCD? 51

How are Brain Structures and Chemicals Related to OCD? 53

   Specific Brain Areas Involved 54

      Basal Ganglia and Amygdala 54

      Pre-frontal and Orbito-frontal Brain Regions 55

   Other Illnesses that Produce OCD-like Symptoms .55

   Neuroimaging Studies in OCD 56

   Biochemical Factors in OCD 59

What are the First-Line Medications Used to Treat OCD? 61

Half-Life and Dosing 63

Effectiveness of SRI Medications for Treating OCD 64

Augmentation Strategies 66

SRI and Antipsychotic Medication Augmentation 66

What Other Medications are Used to Treat OCD? 67

What Other Biologically Based Treatments are Available for OCD? 68

Neurosurgery 68

Electroconvulsive Therapy (ECT) 69

Transcranial Magnetic Stimulation (TMS) 69

Deep Brain Stimulation (DBS) 69

How Effective are Medications vs. Behavior Therapy for Treating OCD? 70

Early (Acute) Treatment Results, Short-term Gains, and Relapse Rates 70

Treatment Compliance 70

Cost Considerations 71

Symptom Types 71

Appendix: Assessment Measures   **73**

Glossary   **77**

References   **83**

Index   **97**

Chapter One:
Overview of Obsessive Compulsive Disorder

This chapter answers the following:

▶ **How Common is OCD?** — This section illustrates the number of people with the disorder and notes differences in OCD between men and women.

▶ **What is the Likelihood of Recovery?** — This section discusses the severity and outcome of the disorder with and without treatment.

O BSESSIVE Compulsive Disorder (OCD) is an anxiety disorder that involves recurrent obsessions or compulsions that are time consuming or cause great difficulty in every day life.[1] Obsessions are recurrent distressing thoughts, images, or impulses that are experienced as unwanted and senseless but difficult, if not impossible, to ignore or resist. Compulsions are behaviors or actions that are often triggered by obsessions. Although countless people with OCD associate a certain life event with the onset of their disorder, many others cannot identify any specific precipitating factors. Common characteristics present in OCD include:

▶ **Obsessional ideas** — Thoughts that intrude into conscious awareness (words, phrases, rhymes) and interfere with the normal flow of thought causing disjointed thinking and emotional distress. The obsessions are often obscene, blasphemous, or nonsensical in content.

▶ **Obsessional images** — Vivid images often depicting violent, sexual, or disturbing scenes (images of a child being killed, cars colliding, excrement, parents engaged in sexual intercourse) that appear repetitively.

▶ **Obsessional convictions** — Beliefs based on irrational assumptions such as "thought equals action" (e.g., thinking ill of my son will cause him to die).

▶ **Obsessional ruminations** — Ponderous worrying (or ritualistic behaviors) (e.g., "Did I lock the door? Turn off the gas?") designed to prevent or alleviate imagined harm or feared consequences.

▶ **Obsessional impulses** — Unwanted impulses related to self-harm (e.g., leaping out of a window), aggression toward others (e.g., smothering a baby), or potentially humiliating behaviors (e.g., shouting obscenities in church).

▶ **Obsessional fears** — Intense anxiety concerning specific objects/items (dirt, disease, animals, blood,

1

etc.) or specific situations/locations (public restrooms, hospitals, etc.), being in a specific situation, or performing particular acts.

▶ **Compulsive rituals** — Repetitive actions (counting, touching, ordering, checking, arranging, cleaning, hoarding, etc.) that produce relief from the obsession.

Written for the professional, this book presents general information about OCD in chapter one, diagnostic information in chapter two, environmental treatments for OCD in chapter three, and medical treatments in chapter four.

How Common is OCD?

Previously considered a very rare mental disorder, OCD now appears to be a hidden epidemic. It is one of the most common mental disorders in the U.S. and is more than twice as prevalent as schizophrenia. Nearly three million Americans suffer from OCD at any given time, with about 7.45 million people (2.5 percent of the population) experiencing OCD symptoms at some point in their lives.[1-4]

OCD symptoms typically begin in late adolescence or early adulthood, with some symptoms beginning possibly in childhood; from one-third to one-half of adult sufferers likely displayed symptoms during childhood.[5-7] Advances in assessment and treatment over the last 20 years have led to an increase in the number of children seeking treatment for OCD.[8, 9] In fact, studies indicate that the incidence of the disorder in children and adolescents up to 18 years of age is anywhere between 0.06 and 2.0 percent.[10, 11] OCD affects men and women of all cultures equally; however, symptoms in children are more frequently observed in boys.[7, 12]

Between one-third and two-thirds of people with OCD have associated significant life events or stresses at the onset of the disorder (e.g., death of a family member, pregnancy, childbirth, or sexual problems).[13] Additional characteristics include indications that:

▶ Slightly more than half of those with OCD are women.[5]

▶ People with OCD have above average intelligence.[14]

▶ Peak age of onset for males is between ages 13 and 15.[5]

▶ Peak age of onset for females is between ages 20 and 24.[5]

▶ Onset usually occurs gradually.

Many people suffering with OCD wait years before seeking treatment. In fact, a survey conducted of patients with OCD revealed an average delay of seven years between the onset of symptoms and the time a patient seeks treatment.[5] This hesitancy to seek treatment may result from shame and embarrassment because people with OCD are often unaware that many others experience similar symptoms.

Ethnic minorities, such as African-Americans, Native Americans, and Asian Americans, often contend with additional obstacles that may further delay identification and treatment of OCD, including a higher level of mistrust of mental health professionals, more reluctance to seek help outside the family or ethnic community, and greater hesitancy to use prescription medications.[15]

Quality of life for those with OCD is generally much worse than for the general population.[16] The severity of OCD ranges from mild (e.g., narrowly focused rituals such as lining up items on one's desk before being able to begin working on a project) to severe (e.g., having to perform a two- or three-hour ritual before being able to go to bed). Many OCD rituals must be completed in a specific sequence, which if interrupted, must be started over from the beginning. These can be particularly crippling as they often consume many hours of the individual's waking day.

Many patients with OCD experience significant functional impairment including job loss, marital disruption, and loss of interpersonal relationships. In fact, the earlier onset of OCD in men may well contribute to their unusually low marriage rate (only 25 percent).[17]

Approximately 50 percent of married individuals with OCD report marital discord resulting from their disorder.[5]

From The Patient's Perspective

I went to a therapist today. I can't stop thinking about awful things that could happen to my husband and my kids. I'm spending more and more time undoing and redoing almost everything I do.

I'm starting to avoid the next task for fear of getting stuck in this pattern all over again. It's starting to affect my relationships and the amount of work I can handle.

What is the Likelihood of Recovery?

Although effective treatments exist, OCD remains a chronic disorder. OCD symptoms routinely vacillate in severity over time and may even disappear completely with or without treatment. Symptom-free intervals are often followed by symptom re-emergence during a time of greater stress or in response to some biological or environmental changes. Long-term studies demonstrate that nine of every 10 individuals with OCD experience a waxing and waning of symptoms, with sustained remissions rare and increases in symptoms often precipitated by stress.[5] While most people with OCD experience considerable symptom fluctuation, as much as 15 percent will follow a deteriorating course with a progressive decline in social and occupational functioning.[1]

Documented recovery rates for individuals suffering from OCD are wide ranging. Estimated rates for spontaneous recovery from OCD range from 25 percent to 71 percent.[12] The highest recovery rates (approximately 90 percent) for OCD are reported after treatment with either behavior therapy or a combination of medication and behavior therapy.[18, 19] In contrast, 60 to 80 percent of those with OCD will improve with medication treatment alone; however, most studies suggest that 70 to 90 percent of patients treated with medication alone will relapse within a few weeks of its discontinuation.[18, 19]

Around 10 percent of individuals with OCD experience distinct periods of OCD symptom exacerbation followed by intervals of relative remission. While the duration of the symptomatic episodes may vary greatly at first — anywhere from several weeks to many months — it typically lengthens as one ages.[5]

Evidence exists that behavior therapy may have more lasting effects. For example, most available evidence suggests that 80 to 90 percent of those with OCD will exhibit noticeable improvement after behavioral therapy, and about 75 percent will maintain symptom improvement on a long-term basis.[5] Although the majority of patients treated with behavior therapy remain improved, as many as 20 to 25 percent will relapse.[5] A bigger obstacle, however, is that up to 25 percent of those with OCD refuse to participate in, or fail to complete, behavior therapy. This resistance is generally attributed to behavior therapy's reliance on exposure techniques, which rely on confronting specific fears in order to conquer them.[5] When this considerable risk of treatment refusal is factored in, the most accurate overall response rate for behavior therapy is more likely around 60 percent, with 10 to 20 percent experiencing no significant reduction in symptoms.

Key Concepts for Chapter One:

1. One-third to two-thirds of those suffering from OCD associate the onset of OCD with a certain life event; others cannot identify any precipitating factor.

2. Nearly three million Americans (2.5 percent of the population) suffer from OCD at any given time.

3. OCD severity ranges from mild (such as ordering/ arranging items) to severe (e.g., performing two- or three-hour rituals before being able to go to bed).

4. Many patients with OCD experience significant functional impairment, including job loss, marital disruption, and loss of relationships.

5. While studies show that behavior therapy has the most lasting effects for patients with OCD, as many as 25 percent of patients refuse to participate in, or fail to complete, behavior therapy.

Chapter Two:
Diagnosing Obsessive Compulsive Disorder

This chapter answers the following:

▶ **What Criteria are Used to Diagnose Obsessive Compulsive Disorder (OCD)?** —This section presents the DSM-IV (TR) diagnostic criteria for OCD.

▶ **What are the Typical Characteristics of Those with OCD?** — This section reviews the primary identifying features of OCD, including avoidance behaviors, excessive guilt, disturbed harm assessment, and excessive worrying.

▶ **What Tools are Available for Clinical Assessment?** — This section provides information on interview processes, self-report instruments, behavioral and psychometric assessments, and laboratory/physical exam findings.

▶ **What Differentiates OCD from Other Disorders?** — This section provides information for differentiating OCD from other disorders.

Behavior rituals are part of our everyday lives, from singing bedtime songs to religious practices to laying out our clothes for the coming day before going to bed. During times of stress, even normal worries can lead to more ritual-like behavior, such as excessive cleaning when a family member is home ill. Diagnosing OCD typically requires the presence of *obsessions* or *compulsions* that persist, make no sense, cause much distress, or interfere with daily functioning. Obsessions are accompanied by uncomfortable feelings, such as fear, disgust, doubt, or a sensation that things have to be done in a way that is "just so." Compulsions differ from compulsive behaviors (e.g., drinking, gambling) in that they do not give the person pleasure; instead they are rituals one performs to get relief from the discomfort they feel over their obsessions. For example, a woman may repeatedly (compulsively) check that she has turned off the stove because she is obsessed with the thought that she might accidentally burn down her house.

obsessions — thoughts, images, or impulses that occur over and over again and feel out of one's control

compulsions — acts the person performs over and over again, often according to certain "rules"

What Criteria are Used to Diagnose Obsessive Compulsive Disorder (OCD)?

Diagnosing OCD can be tricky because superstitions, rituals, or other behaviors can resemble OCD symptoms. This chapter discusses how to differentiate those behaviors from OCD, reviews the diagnostic criteria and key characteristics of the disorder, and covers various tools available for clinical assessment.

*The main criteria for diagnosing OCD (see figure 2.1 on the following page) comes from the leading psychiatric diagnostic manual used in the United States, the **Diagnostic and Statistical Manual of Mental Disorders, Fourth Edition, Text Revision,** published by the American Psychiatric Association.*

Figure 2.1 DSM-IV(TR) Criteria for Obsessive Compulsive Disorder

I. 300.3 Obsessive-Compulsive Disorder

A. Either obsessions or compulsions:

Obsessions as defined by (1), (2), (3), and (4):

1. recurrent and persistent thoughts, impulses, or images that are experienced, at some time during the disturbance, as intrusive and inappropriate and that cause marked anxiety or distress

2. the thoughts, impulses, or images are not simply excessive worries about real-life problems

3. the person attempts to ignore or suppress such thoughts, impulses, or images, or to neutralize them with some other thought or action

4. the person recognizes that the obsessional thoughts, impulses, or images are a product of his or her own mind (not imposed from without as in thought insertion)

Compulsions as defined by (1) and (2):

1. repetitive behaviors (e.g., hand washing, ordering, checking) or mental acts (e.g., praying, counting, repeating words silently) that the person feels driven to perform in response to an obsession, or according to rules that must be applied rigidly

2. the behaviors or mental acts are aimed at preventing or reducing distress or preventing some dreaded event or situation; however, these behaviors or mental acts either are not connected in a realistic way with what they are designed to neutralize or prevent or are clearly excessive

B. At some point during the course of the disorder, the person has recognized that the obsessions or compulsions are excessive or unreasonable. **Note:** This does not apply to children.

C. The obsessions or compulsions cause marked distress, are time consuming (take more than 1 hour a day), or significantly interfere with the person's normal routine, occupational (or academic) functioning, or usual social activities or relationships.

D. If another Axis I disorder is present, the content of the obsessions or compulsions is not restricted to it (e.g., preoccupation with food in the presence of an Eating Disorder; hair pulling in the presence of Trichotillomania; concern with appearance in the presence of Body Dysmorphic Disorder; preoccupation with drugs in the presence of a Substance Use Disorder; preoccupation with having a serious illness in the presence of Hypochondriasis; preoccupation with sexual urges or fantasies in the presence of a Paraphilia; or guilty ruminations in the presence of Major Depressive Disorder).

E. The disturbance is not due to the direct physiological effects of a substance (e.g., a drug of abuse, a medication) or a general medical condition.

Specify if:

With Poor Insight: if, for most of the time during the current episode, the person does not recognize that the obsessions and compulsions are excessive or unreasonable

(Reprinted with permission by the American Psychiatric Association: *Diagnostic and Statistical Manual of Mental Disorders, Fourth Edition, Text Revision*, Washington, D.C., American Psychiatric Association, 2000).[1]

What are the Typical Characteristics of Those with OCD?

Those who suffer from OCD may have only a few or suffer from many typical symptoms. These symptoms distress the individual and often cause problems in the work place and in personal relationships. In rare instances, OCD may leave a person house-bound when the sufferer's fears and worries make it easier to stay home in perceived relative safety rather than risk facing situations that may trigger their OCD. Common features of OCD include:

- **Avoiding feared situations/stimuli related to obsessions** — Those with OCD may experience the need to avoid a variety of feared situations or stimuli, to the point of making extreme life-style changes to do so. For example, obsessive fears related to dirt or contamination result in avoidance of public restrooms or shaking hands with strangers.

- **Overestimating the importance of thoughts and having a pathological sense of responsibility** — Those with OCD often experience guilt and fear that their thoughts might cause harm to others or make something terrible happen, because many individuals with OCD believe that having a thought is the same as actually acting on that thought. Further, many people with OCD perform compulsions because they believe that failing to "correct" a problem is equivalent to caus-ing it. Their compulsions are a way of undoing or fixing something they fear they may have done wrong or some-thing that might result in harm to others (e.g., removing a rock from the road so that a car does not subsequently hit it and have an accident).[20]

- **Overestimating harm** — Another OCD characteristic is a tendency to overestimate both the likelihood of harm and the severity of the consequences.[21] Those with OCD may assume that an environment is dangerous until proven safe. This contrasts sharply with a common presumption that all is well unless danger is obvious.

- **Worrying and ruminating excessively** — Anxious individuals may find themselves frequently thinking about personal and/or family concerns that may or may not be linked to obsessions. Such individuals may use *sedatives* excessively to try to combat their symptoms. They may also try to control their fears by using alcohol or *hypnotics*.

sedatives — medications that help suppress anxiety by calming agitation and relaxing muscles

hypnotics — medications that promote sleep

What Tools are Available for Clinical Assessment?

Clinical assessment involves gathering specific information from: clinical interviews, self-report instruments and structured interviews, behavioral assessments, psychometric assessments, and laboratory/physical exam findings.

Clinical Interviews

During the clinical interview, the clinician gathers information about obsessive cues and rituals, medical history, individual and family psychiatric history, social and occupational functioning, the role of relatives, and patient insight.

In addition to questions of history and current functioning, the interviewer inquires about:

- ▶ External sources of obsessive fear (e.g., seeing lights on, touching a doorknob, reading about AIDS, or hearing news about a hit-and-run accident)
- ▶ Internal cues, including thoughts, images, impulses, and feared consequences of not performing compulsions
- ▶ Avoidance behavior (e.g., not driving because of fear of running over a pedestrian)[18, 22]

Medical History

An initial evaluation of an individual presenting with OCD symptoms should always include a comprehensive medical evaluation. Several medical and/or neurological conditions including infections, toxins, brain lesions, or injury can produce OCD symptoms presumably by disruption of the same brain structures implicated in the development of the disorder. OCD cannot be diagnosed in individuals who develop symptoms secondary to infection, lesions, or acute brain injury or illness as the treatment, course, and prognosis for individuals with OCD due to a general medical condition is markedly different.[23–31] Medical conditions associated with the development of OCD symptoms include:

- ▶ Brain tumor or abnormal blood vessels
- ▶ Brain injury, infection or disease such as:
    - ▶ Injury to brain, causing *anoxia* (lack of oxygen)
    - ▶ Toxic exposure (carbon monoxide poisoning or manganese intoxication)
    - ▶ Brain infection, such as viral *encephalitis* that may result in *post-encephalitic Parkinsonism*
    - ▶ Bacterial infection that spreads to the brain [*Sydenham's chorea* or pediatric autoimmune

anoxia — brain cell death resulting from interruption of oxygen supply to the brain

encephalitis — viral infection of the brain leading to inflammation

Post-encephalitic Parkinsonism — rigidity, tremor, and abnormally slow movements that develop as a result of encephalitis lethargica or "sleeping sickness"

Sydenham's chorea — rheumatic fever that spreads into the brain and damages the basal ganglion, resulting in involuntary, irregular (choreo-athetoid) muscle movements of the face, neck, and limbs

neuropsychiatric disorders associated with streptococcal infections (*PANDAS*)]

▶ Degenerative brain disease, such as Parkinson's disease, *progressive supranuclear palsy*, Huntington's chorea, multiple sclerosis, or dementia

▶ General medical illnesses, such as:

  ▶ Diabetes mellitus

  ▶ Thyroid impairment

▶ Substance abuse (including overuse of prescribed medications) such as:

  ▶ Amphetamines or stimulants (methamphetamine, crank, speed)

  ▶ Cocaine or crack

  ▶ Diet pills

  ▶ Hallucinogens (LSD, "acid," ecstasy, MDMA)

▶ Developmental or learning disorders such as:

  ▶ Mental retardation

  ▶ Autism, Asperger's syndrome

▶ Other psychiatric conditions, such as:

  ▶ Depression with psychotic features

  ▶ Other anxiety disorders, such as panic disorder, generalized anxiety disorder, social anxiety disorder, agoraphobia, or post-traumatic stress disorder

▶ Psychotic disorders, such as delusional disorders or schizophrenia

▶ Somatization disorders such as *body dysmorphic disorder*, hypochondriasis

▶ Impulse control disorders such as *trichotillomania*, compulsive gambling

Individual and Family Psychiatric History

An individual psychiatric history should include questions on:

▶ The age of onset of OCD symptoms

▶ Severity and pattern of symptoms (episodic versus persistent)

▶ Significant stresses (psychosocial and medical)

▶ Evidence of depression, other psychiatric illness, or personality disorder

These factors may impact the treatment plan and ultimately the long-term prognosis for an individual with OCD. For example, severe symptoms without an associated significant stressor and accompanied by evidence of *schizotypal personality disorder*

PANDAS — complication of untreated strep throat where the streptococcus bacteria invades the brain in children/adolescents and results in damage to the basal ganglia region, producing OCD symptoms

progressive supranuclear palsy — genetic/familial condition characterized by deterioration of the brain cells in the cerebral cortex, basal ganglia, and other upper motor areas and resulting in weakness and/or paralysis

For more information on distinguishing OCD from other disorders, see pages 15–19.

body dysmorphic disorder — a mental disorder that involves a disturbed body image

trichotillomania — a disorder characterized by a repeated urge to pull out scalp, facila, or body hair as well as eyelashes

schizotypal personality disorder — a personality disorder characterized by markedly eccentric and erratic thought, speech, and behavior as well as a tendency to withdraw from other people suggest a poor prognosis.[32] Such conditions may necessitate long-term therapy as well as medication interventions. On the other hand, mild symptoms, an identifiable significant stressor, and lack of a personality disorder, suggest a very favorable treatment outlook. Brief behavioral interventions may be sufficient for the symptoms to go into remission.

Family and genetic histories provide clues about OCD diagnosis. Patient assessment and initial screening should include questions about family psychiatric history, especially the presence of *Tourette's syndrome* in relatives, since Tourette's is more common in families of those with OCD.[1]

Tourette's syndrome — neurological disorder characterized by semi-voluntary motor tics and vocalizations

Social and Occupational Functioning

Collecting a social and occupational history will help identify any functional impairment required to diagnose OCD. Clinicians should ask about school or job performance, socializing, and status of friendships and intimate relationships. To diagnose OCD, obsessions and compulsions must consume at least one hour per day and cause marked distress or significant interference in a person's routine, occupational functioning, and/or usual social activities and relationships. Therefore, a clinician must determine if these criteria are met using questions, such as:

- ▶ How much time per day do you spend obsessing and ritualizing?
- ▶ Have your symptoms caused you much distress?
- ▶ Have your obsessions and compulsions interfered with your occupational or academic functioning, causing you to lose jobs or drop out of school?
- ▶ Have your symptoms interfered with your functioning in social or family situations?
- ▶ Have your symptoms caused marked distress in your social activities or relationships?

Based on the answers to these questions, the clinician first determines whether or not the criteria for OCD have been met. If so, the clinician assesses the severity and pervasiveness of the symptoms. The more severe the symptoms and the occupational and social impairment, the poorer the treatment *prognosis*. Patients with OCD who have moderate symptoms and modest or relatively recent impairments in occupational and social functioning respond best to behavioral interventions.

prognosis — outcome in the future

Role of Relatives

Because family members' attitudes and responses have been found to predict treatment outcome, the clinician must determine the role of relatives. Family members who are emotionally overinvolved or hostile to the patient negatively influence treatment outcome and predict higher rates of treatment dropout.[33, 34]

Family involvement in the patient's rituals may interfere with successful treatment, making early identification of this obstacle essential. Family participation in and accommodation for the patient's rituals is highly related to:[35, 36]

► Greater family dysfunction

► Family distress

► Rejection of the patient with OCD by family members

► Increased severity of OCD symptoms in the patient

Alternately, non-hostile criticism from family members appears to improve treatment outcomes for patients with OCD.[36]

Patient Insight

Those who perceive their obsessions and compulsions as irrational have a better treatment prognosis.[37] According to changes in the DSM-IV (TR), however, OCD may still be diagnosed even though the individual fails to recognize the irrationality of his or her obsessions or compulsions during episodes. DSM-IV (TR) designates these individuals as, "With Poor Insight."[1] However, DSM-IV (TR) does specify that adults with OCD must comprehend that their obsessions or compulsions are excessive or unreasonable at some point during the course of the disorder. Patients who have poor insight and overestimate the likelihood of harm are less likely to benefit from behavior therapy but may be helped by medications.[38] However, those treated with a combination of cognitive-behavioral therapy and medications may experience increased insight.[39]

Self-Report Instruments and Structured Interviews

There are two general classes of instruments used to detect and diagnose OCD. The first includes self-report instruments completed by patients to either screen for OCD in various settings or to classify subjects for research purposes. For example:

► Obsessive Compulsive Inventory-Short Version (OCI-SV)

► Padua Inventory (PI)

► Compulsive Activity Checklist (CAC)

► Yale-Brown Obsessive Compulsive Checklist and Scale (Y-BOCS) — Self-report Version

► Vancouver Obsessional Compulsive Inventory (VOCI)

The second class of instruments includes structured interviews in which trained clinicians follow a strict interview format to probe for OCD diagnosis and severity.

A recent study found that 75 percent of relatives of persons with OCD were participating at least minimally in rituals, avoidance, or modifying their own behavior to accommodate the patients' symptoms.[33]

Most people with OCD know that (between episodes) their fears and rituals are irrational; however, they may lose this insight in the face of their obsessional cues. These patients are much more likely to benefit from behavior therapy and medications than those who are continually convinced of the accuracy of their obsessive fears.

These instruments are covered in detail in the appendix.

The VOCI is an updated version of the Maudsley Obsessional Compulsive Inventory (MOCI), which has been widely used for measuring observable OCD behaviors such as washing and checking.

These instruments are covered in detail in the appendix.

These instruments include:

► Structured Clinical Interview for DSM-IV (SCID)

► Anxiety Disorders Interview Schedule (ADIS)

► Yale-Brown Obsessive Compulsive Scale (Y-BOCS) and Symptom Checklist — Interview Version

Based on a recent analysis of factors evaluated with the PI (as self-report instrument) and the Y-BOCS (clinician-rated version), researchers recommend using both instruments to assess the full spectrum of OCD symptoms as both widely used inventories have unique factors.[40]

Behavior Assessment

Behavioral avoidance tests (BAT) were originally developed to measure fear and avoidance in people with phobias.[41] Several types of BATs have been used to assess obsessive-compulsive symptoms. A single-task BAT involves presenting the patient with a feared stimulus, perhaps a garbage can. The clinician asks the patient to approach as close as possible to the object and report his or her level of discomfort on a 100-point *Subjective Units of Distress (SUDs) scale*. The clinician measures avoidance behavior in terms of the SUDs scale and the patient's distance from the feared object or willingness to engage in sequential exposure steps.

Subjective Units of Distress (SUDs) scale — a scale ranging from 10–100 with 10 being the least anxiety provoking and 100 being the most anxiety provoking. The SUDs scoring system allows the patient to express exactly how upsetting or distressing certain stimuli are in comparison to other anxiety experiences.

Because a single-task BAT may fail to capture the range of an individual's obsessive-compulsive symptoms, multi-task BATs are needed for most patients. In this approach, the clinician has patients repeat the avoidance test with several different objects or situations that represent the range of their fears. BATs provide "real-life" measures of fear and avoidance in OCD and are well suited for assessing fear and avoidance of "contaminated" stimuli associated with washing compulsions. However, BATs

From The Patient's Perspective

Saw Owen today. She asked a lot of questions and said she'd help me get things back under control. I know I'm unreasonably worried about my family, so I've tried to stop doing everything over and over so much. It's all so depressing, and I'm so tired. Owen says I have to fill out this questionnaire that asks all these questions about how often I do things and how I think and feel. I hope this is worth all the trouble!

may be more difficult to apply in cases of checking, repeating, or ordering compulsions. Another problem with BATs is that a patient's fear and avoidance may be situation-specific. The patient with OCD may fear and avoid touching objects at home yet handle objects fearlessly in other environments. In these cases, conduct a BAT at home or in whatever environment symptoms emerge.

One study supports the use of an in-home BAT for assessing treatment-related changes in children and adolescents with OCD.[42]

Psychometric Assessments

In inpatient and outpatient settings, clinicians regularly use *psychometric instruments* to facilitate diagnosis and describe patient personality characteristics. Although these instruments are not specific to patients with OCD, they may provide clinicians with useful information. Commonly used psychometric instruments are:

psychometric instruments — tests that measure psychological factors, such as personality, intelligence, beliefs, and fears

- ► Minnesota Multiphasic Personality Inventories (MMPI and MMPI-2)
- ► Rorschach Inkblot Test
- ► Thematic Apperception Test (TAT)
- ► Wechsler Adult Intelligence Scale-III (WAIS-III)

Laboratory/Physical Exam Findings

Laboratory findings, although helpful in continued research regarding the cause or effects of OCD on human physiology, do not appear to add precision to diagnostic decisions. There are no laboratory findings specific to an OCD diagnosis; however, patients may exhibit skin disorders caused by excessive washing with water or with harsh cleaning agents.[1]

What Differentiates OCD from Other Disorders?

When diagnosing OCD, the clinician must rule out the possibility that the patient's symptoms are related to:

People with OCD do not enjoy participating in their compulsions. They would gladly give up these behaviors if they did not have to experience the anxiety that happens whenever they try to stop the rituals.

- ► Addictive disorders
- ► Anxiety disorder due to a general medical condition
- ► Body dysmorphic disorder
- ► Delusional disorder or psychotic disorder not otherwise specified
- ► Generalized anxiety disorder, panic disorder, or post-traumatic stress disorder
- ► Hypochondriasis
- ► Major depressive episode (or mood disorder)

- ▶ Obsessive compulsive personality disorder
- ▶ Phobias
- ▶ Schizophrenia
- ▶ Substance-induced anxiety disorder
- ▶ Superstitions and repetitive checking behaviors
- ▶ Tics or Tourette's syndrome

Addictive Disorders

Although labeled "compulsive," addictive behaviors (e.g., excessive eating, sexual behavior, gambling, or substance use) are unlike OCD compulsions. People performing impulsive behaviors, such as gambling, usually derive pleasure from the activity. They wish to resist it only because of harmful consequences, such as losing all their money. In contrast, individuals with OCD perform compulsions to reduce anxiety by avoiding some imagined negative consequence (e.g., someone having an accident or a house burning down).

Anxiety Disorder Due to a General Medical Condition

To ensure appropriate treatment, the clinician needs to determine if the anxiety or obsessive compulsive symptoms are related to or caused by a primary medical condition. A physician can use medical history, laboratory findings, or physical examination to rule out that possibility.[1]

General medical conditions that may cause anxiety include:

pheochromocytoma — a ususally benign tumor that causes increased secretion of epinephrine or norepinephrine

- ▶ Endocrine problems, such as: hyperthyroidism, hypothyroidism, *pheochromocytoma,* hypoglycemia, or hyperglycemia (diabetes)
- ▶ Cardiac problems, such as: heart failure or arrhythmia (irregular heart beat)
- ▶ Pulmonary problems, such as: chronic obstructive pulmonary disease (emphysema, asthma), embolism, pneumonia, or hyperventilation

porphyria — a disorder involving the metabolism of phrphyrin — the foundation structure of hemoglobin, chlorophyll, and certain enzymes

- ▶ Nutritional problems, such as: vitamin B12 deficiency or *porphyria*
- ▶ Other conditions, such as: neoplasms (tumors, cancer) or encephalitis

Body Dysmorphic Disorder

Recurrent or intrusive thoughts, images, or behaviors often occur in the context of other mental disorders. The clinician should not diagnose OCD if the content of the patient's thoughts or activities is exclusively related to another mental disorder. For instance, a preoccupation with appearance accompanied by an irrational fear of having a physical defect, and related checking rituals would be diagnosed as body dysmorphic disorder.

Delusional Disorder or Psychotic Disorder Not Otherwise Specified

A person's ability to realize that obsessions or compulsions are excessive or irrational occurs on a continuum. In some individuals with OCD, reality testing may be absent, and the obsession may reach delusional proportions (e.g., actually believing that one caused a plane to crash by having willed it). In such cases, the presence of psychotic features may warrant an additional diagnosis of delusional disorder or psychotic disorder not otherwise specified. The specifier, "With Poor Insight," may be helpful in situations that are on the boundary between obsession and delusion. For example, a patient with OCD who realizes most of the time that they are not responsible for plane crashes but occasionally worries that they really might have caused one, would be diagnosed as having OCD with poor insight.

> OCD can be diagnosed concurrently with a psychotic disorder when criteria for both disorders are met.

Generalized Anxiety Disorder, Panic Disorder, or Post-Traumatic Stress Disorder

The worries experienced by those with generalized anxiety disorder (GAD) are excessive and persistent concerns about real-life circumstances. In contrast, those with OCD experience obsessions whose content is more likely to be unrealistic and seen by the patient as inappropriate.[5] For example, persistent but fairly rational worries about finances, health concerns, or one's job would be considered GAD, whereas irrational fears of causing a fire by leaving the stove on or harming one's child with a knife constitute obsessions.

> The presence of rituals is unique to OCD. For example, a person with generalized anxiety disorder (GAD) may worry constantly about having enough money to pay their bills. However, they will not repetitively count their money or call the bank to check on their deposits.

The hallmark of panic disorder is the presence of spontaneous, unprovoked panic attacks. While certain thoughts or stimuli (e.g., germs), can precipitate anxiety attacks that resemble panic in OCD, patients do not experience unprovoked anxiety. Instead, intrusive images or certain stimuli trigger anxiety in OCD.

Recurrent images or flashbacks can occur during post-traumatic stress disorder (PTSD), but these symptoms emerge after a life-threatening event or tragedy that has already occurred. In OCD, the intrusive thoughts or excessive fears concern things that might happen.

Hypochondriasis

Hypochondriasis should be diagnosed instead of OCD if persistent, distressing thoughts are exclusively related to fears of a serious illness despite considerable evidence (reassurances from physicians, normal test results, etc.) to the contrary. While individuals with OCD may worry about and seek medical help for multiple, presumed physical symptoms or diseases, they realize their concerns are excessive. However, if the concern about having a disease is focused on one medical condition (such as cancer) and is followed by rituals, such as excessive washing or checking the body, then OCD may be considered as an alternative diagnosis or added as a secondary diagnosis to hypochondriasis.

Major Depressive Episode

Major depressive episode and OCD occur concurrently in 30 to 35 percent of people with OCD seeking treatment. If all other criteria for OCD are met, symptoms of sleep disturbance, isolation, and brooding resulting from obsessions and compulsions would indicate an OCD diagnosis rather than a major depressive episode.

Ruminations are common in depressed individuals and develop as part of a depressed mood. They tend to resolve with effective treatment of the depression. Unlike individuals with OCD who attempt to ignore or suppress obsessions, people with depression do not typically try to suppress or ignore their depressive brooding.[5]

Both OCD and major depression often involve symptoms of isolation and sleep disturbance. However, it is the source of these disturbances, rather than the disturbance itself, that differentiates depression from OCD. For example, a sleep disturbance caused by obsessional worry that one has caused a catastrophe would be related to OCD, while sleep disturbance accompanied by a sense of despair and hopelessness would signify depression.

Obsessive Compulsive Personality Disorder

People with OCPD do not usually complain of anxiety.

Although the names, "OCD" and "Obsessive-Compulsive Personality Disorder (OCPD)" are similar, clinical presentations is quite different. OCPD does not involve the presence of true obsessions or compulsions. Instead, it involves a pervasive pattern of preoccupation with orderliness, perfectionism, rigid rules, and control at the expense of flexibility and openness. Individuals with OCPD do not clean or check things fearing a resulting tragedy. Rather, they simply require order, perfection, and control in their lives. Hoarding or excessive collecting of possessions can be a symptom of OCPD or OCD. If an individual expresses symptoms of both disorders, the clinician can make a dual diagnosis.

Phobias

Patients with OCD may avoid the same situations as those with agoraphobia; however, their responses are often due to fears of contamination or acting on unwanted or aggressive impulses.

Agoraphobia is characterized by a person's fear of being in a situation that causes him or her to have an anxiety attack. Typically, these include being in crowded places or on bridges, traveling away from home, and similar situations where the person feels unable to escape.

A preoccupation limited to a feared object (e.g., snakes) or situation would be diagnosed as a specific or *social phobia*. An additional diagnosis of OCD may be warranted if there are obsessions or compulsions whose content is not related to the other mental disorder. Specific phobia of illness should be diagnosed instead of OCD if the patient's primary worry involves contracting an illness (rather than having an illness) and no rituals are involved.[5]

social phobia — a disorder characterized by episodes of panic anxiety in social settings, due to excessive concern about public embarrassment or possible adverse scrutiny

Schizophrenia

Like some schizophrenic delusions, the content of OCD obsessions may be quite bizarre, such as the belief that one might accidentally seal one's self into an envelope and get deposited into a mailbox.[5] The difference is that those with OCD are aware of the irrational nature of these fears. They typically do not show other symptoms of psychosis or schizophrenia, such as: marked *loosening of associations*, prominent *hallucinations*, grossly *inappropriate affect, or thought insertion*.

loosening of associations — an individual's speech slips off the track from one topic to another

hallucinations — false sensory perceptions

inappropriate affect — mood incongruent with context of a situation

thought insertion — the belief that some other being is placing thoughts in one's mind

Substance-Induced Anxiety Disorder

A substance-induced anxiety disorder diagnosis involves excessive anxiety judged by the clinician as directly related to the physiological effect of abusing a substance, side effects of a prescribed or over-the-counter medication, or toxin exposure. Clinicians can differentiate this disorder from OCD by using careful history (and perhaps a urine drug screen) to determine if OCD symptoms were triggered by use of or cessation from an illicit substance, alcohol, or a medication.[1]

Symptoms of substance-induced anxiety disorder may be associated with either use or cessation of both prescription and nonprescription drugs.

Superstitions and Repetitive Checking Behaviors

Superstitious behaviors, although frequently encountered in everyday life, lead to a diagnosis of OCD only if these behaviors are elaborated repetitively, appear to have obsessive content (e.g., magical thinking that triggers rituals, consuming more than one hour per day), and result in clinically significant impairment or distress.

Tics

In contrast to compulsions, tics are sudden, rapid, recurrent, non-rhythmic, stereotyped motor movements or vocalizations (e.g., eye blinking, tongue protrusion, or throat clearing), which are often performed in response to sensations of subjective discomfort. Tics are not aimed at neutralizing an obsession or preventing an unwanted outcome. Some people have both OCD and a tic disorder (especially Tourette's syndrome).

Key Concepts for Chapter Two:

1. Patients with OCD may experience only a few or many of the typical symptoms of the illness, including: avoiding feared situations, having a pathological sense of responsibility, fearing they may cause harm to others, overestimating harm, and worrying/ ruminating excessively.

2. Medical conditions and family psychiatric history can impact the treatment plan and the long-term prognosis for patients with OCD.

3. Clinicians must determine the family dynamics that could negatively affect treatment (such as family members' participation in rituals and avoidance behavior), as well as identify family members who may be able to assist in treatment.

4. Researchers recommend using both self-report instruments (e.g., the Padua Inventory) and clinician-rated instruments (e.g., the Yale-Brown Obsessive Compulsive Scale — interview version) to assess the full spectrum of OCD symptoms.

5. Those with OCD may present "with poor insight," meaning that they sometimes fail to realize that their obsessions or compulsions are excessive or irrational.

6. It is important to distinguish OCD from other disorders such as generalized anxiety disorder, in which fears relate to real-life circumstances and are excessive and persistent. Those with OCD suffer from more unrealistic fears.

Chapter Three:
Psychosocial Treatments for Obsessive Compulsive Disorder

This chapter answers the following:

► **What Social and Psychological Influences May Cause Obsessive Compulsive Disorder (OCD)?** — This section presents various theoretical approaches to understanding OCD from a psychological perspective. These include behavioral, cognitive, and psychodynamic theories as well as group and family therapy approaches.

► **What is the Behavior Therapy Approach to Treating OCD?** — This section reviews early as well as more recent behavioral treatment methods, especially exposure and response prevention and treatment efficacy.

► **What is the Cognitive Therapy Approach to Treating OCD?** — This section focuses on rational emotive therapy and Beck's cognitive therapy as well as efficacy research.

► **What is the Psychoanalytic Approach to Treating OCD?** — This section reviews psychoanalytic theories, treatment methods, and efficacy.

► **What is the Group Therapy Approach to Treating OCD?** — This section reviews treatment methods and efficacy for psychoeducational and behavioral group approaches.

► **What is the Family Therapy Approach to Treating OCD?** — This section reviews family therapy approaches and efficacy.

OR decades, researchers have searched for the origin of OCD. Unfortunately, while successful treatments suggest possible causes of OCD, the exact *etiology* remains unknown. Because both psychological and biological treatment studies indicate similar results and because combining these treatments is effective, some researchers suggest that questioning whether or not OCD has a single origin is outdated.[25] The most accurate answer to the question of OCD's etiology is that psychological, biological, and environmental factors are involved in the disorder's etiology.

etiology — the cause of a disorder

Recent research indicates that both behavioral and medication treatments produce similar beneficial changes in brain function; demonstrating that the psychology and biology of OCD are interrelated. This research indicates that successful behavior therapy results in similar changes or adaptations in the underlying function of certain brain areas that occur after effective medication therapy. Specifically, after 10 weeks of treatment with behavior therapy or *serotonergic medication*, approximately the same number of patients improved in both groups. In the improved patients, no matter what method of treatment was used, the previously hyperactive areas in the brain returned to normal.

serotonergic medication — medications that specifically affect the neurotransmitter serotonin

21

Though the treatments seem very different, they may ultimately achieve success through the same mechanisms.[43–45]

This chapter explores environmental influences that may cause OCD and reviews corresponding psychological interventions. Chapter four explores biological theories, including the *serotonin hypothesis*, that suggest that certain brain regions and the underlying transmission of the neurotransmitter serotonin may cause or mediate OCD symptoms. Chapter four also explores in detail the effectiveness of using medications and psychotherapy individually and in combination.

What Social and Psychological Influences May Cause OCD?

Many theorists believe that environment and life experiences play a major role in OCD's origin. There are numerous theories regarding the environmental causes and individual treatments of OCD. This section examines the following:

► **Behavioral theories and treatments** — These theories emphasize a learned pattern of fear and avoidance behavior in response to a certain stimulus or situation. For example, an individual may refuse to use public lavatories due to an intense fear of being contaminated by germs. The behavioral model focuses on how individuals acquire obsessions by learning to associate a neutral event with fear. The individual then attempts to cope with that fear or anxiety by performing compulsive rituals reinforced because they temporarily reduce this anxiety. Behavioral treatments are based on *habituation* of anxiety and/or distress when the patient confronts feared situations.

► **Cognitive theories and treatments** — These theories propose that expectations and beliefs about threat, control, and responsibility influence anxious responses to previously neutral stimuli. For example, an individual may feel responsible for an intrusive thought about harming others impulsively and thus may repeatedly check while driving to be sure he or she has not hit a pedestrian. Cognitive models focus on how an individual's perceptions, internal thoughts, images, and belief systems affect behavior when experiencing an intrusive (obsessive) idea. Treatment methods employ techniques to promote rational thinking and tend to incorporate behavioral strategies because of the interplay between cognitions and behavior.

serotonin hypothesis — the theory that impaired serotonin neurotransmission in the brain relates to OCD development

The multidimensional nature of OCD's origin has brought about distinct treatment models. These models are based on theories that specifically focus on psychological origins as well as those theories suggesting a neurophysiological origin.

See pages 23–31 for a complete discussion of behavioral treatment methods and effectiveness.

habituation — gradual, naturally occurring reduction of anxiety or discomfort over time, if exposure is maintained

See pages 32–37 for a complete discussion of cognitive treatment methods.

▶ **Psychoanalytic theories and treatments** — The psychoanalytic model assumes that both personal history and early development interact to determine:

  ▶ An individual's personality

  ▶ Coping styles that may increase vulnerability for psychological problems, such as OCD

Treatment methods focus on identifying early life events and family relationships affecting present emotions and behavior that contribute to OCD symptoms.

See pages 37–39 for a complete discussion of psychoanalytic treatment methods.

▶ **Group and family treatments** — Group and family therapies focus on the interpersonal aspects of the development of and the improvement in OCD symptoms. These treatments are based mainly on behavioral methods using group and family assistants to encourage patient cooperation.

See pages 39–48 for a complete discussion of group and family treatment methods.

What is the Behavior Therapy Approach to Treating OCD?

In general, behavior theory and treatment focus on how behavior is learned and how it can be unlearned. Treatment models for behavior therapy stem from a two-stage theory for the acquisition and maintenance of fear and avoidance behavior.[5] According to this theory, a neutral object, (e.g., a knife or toilet) or thought (e.g., an image of the devil or the number "13") first becomes associated with fear by being paired with an anxiety-provoking stimulus (e.g., fear of contamination or an image of harming someone else). To reduce the anxiety developed, patients use escape or avoidance responses that are repeated and reinforced because they initially decrease anxiety.

Behavior clinicians believe that obsessions give rise to anxiety, and compulsions temporarily reduce that anxiety.[2] Individuals with OCD use compulsive rituals to actively reduce distress because what triggers obsessions is so prominent that it cannot be passively avoided. For example, individuals wash their hands dozens of times daily because they cannot avoid dirt and germs entirely.

Behavioral Treatment Methods

Based on the theory that obsessions evoke anxiety or discomfort, which is then reduced by compulsions, early behavioral theorists believed that OCD treatment should include anxiety-reducing procedures and a way to block the reinforcement embedded in the emission of rituals. This section reviews these early behavioral treatments, which led to the more current treatment methods: imagined exposure, in-vivo exposure, and response prevention. This section also addresses common concerns about exposure and response prevention and presents research on the effectiveness of behavioral treatments with OCD.

Early Behavioral Treatments

Early behavioral treatments focused on reducing the anxiety associated with obsessions. Practitioners believed that once obsessional cues ceased to evoke anxiety, compulsive behavior would stop because it was no longer reinforced by its anxiety-reducing properties. For example, once a person no longer felt so anxious at the thought of being contaminated, he or she would reduce or stop excessive cleaning rituals. Clinicians expected these anxiety-reducing treatments to make the patient more comfortable in anxiety-eliciting situations by using prolonged exposure. This mental or physical exposure also breaks the connection between the anxiety-producing stimulus and feared disaster because exposure fails to result in disaster. Patients' expectations of negative consequences are not reinforced, and they adopt new, more rational expectations when faced with the previously anxiety-producing situation. Some of the early anxiety-reducing treatments for OCD, most of which proved to be of little help, included:[46]

systematic desensitization — a clinical technique that pairs relaxation with imagery of anxiety-eliciting situations

▶ *Systematic desensitization* — This procedure consists of inducing a state of relaxation in the patient and then presenting anxiety-evoking items arranged in a hierarchical order. Clinicians believed that the pairing of relaxation with the disturbing stimuli would wear down (habituate) associated anxiety.

paradoxical intention — a technique where the clinician instructs the patient to do more of the obsessions or compulsions

▶ *Paradoxical intention* — This treatment involves deliberate attempts to increase the frequency or intensity of obsessions or compulsions to reduce discomfort.[43] For example, a clinician asks a patient to deliberately think about germs and needing to wash more than usual

From The Patient's Perspective

Jim's getting tired of my crazy stuff, and I can't blame him. Owen wants to talk to both of us together about behavior therapy. It scares me, but I've got to do something. She says I might feel less afraid if my depression improves.

She also recommended medication for my depression before starting behavior therapy.

because the danger from germs is so great. The clinician then assigns homework based on this scenario.

▶ *Imagined flooding* — Imagined flooding usually involves the clinician encouraging the patient to mentally experience their fears during the therapy session. For example, a patient who compulsively checks things might be asked to visualize leaving the house without checking any locks and experiencing what that would feel like. The clinician might also ask the patient to visualize a feared outcome, such as being robbed.

▶ *Satiation* — Satiation focuses on verbal repetition. For example, a patient fearful that repeating certain words or phrases would lead to his mother's death might be asked to repeatedly discuss those fears in great detail with the help of the clinician. The verbalized obsession might also be tape recorded for playback as homework. Additional early behavioral treatments, such as *aversion relief* and *thought stopping,* were aimed at blocking obsessions and compulsions.

Aversion relief involved the act of punishing an undesired behavior or ritual and stopping the punishment when the undesired behavior stopped. For example, a clinician might make electric shock contingent on doing a ritual, such as hand washing. The clinician would then stop the shock as soon as the person touched a contaminated object. Therefore, patients experienced discomfort when they performed a ritual and relief when they touched feared objects, the reverse of their usual pattern. This method can also be applied to mental rituals so that the person experiences relief when no longer engaging in obsessive thoughts. In effect, the shock reciprocally inhibits the problematic rituals due to its aversive nature. This treatment is intended to teach the patient to resist rituals even in the face of obsession-eliciting stimuli.[46]

The process of thought stopping aims to prohibit obsessions by replacing them with more pleasant and calming thoughts. It involves disrupting obsessional thoughts through the use of a cue word, like "Stop!" The clinician teaches the patient to utilize this cue word when experiencing unwanted obsessional thoughts. In addition, the clinician instructs the patient to visualize a pleasant scene immediately after saying the cue word. For example, a clinician would teach an individual who always fears hitting someone while driving to say, "Stop!" when the thought that he or she has hit someone arises. Immediately after saying "Stop," the patient pictures a happy and pleasant scene. The patient decides what scene to imagine (e.g., a sunny day on a tropical beach or a beautiful cabin on a lake in the mountains).

imagined flooding — a clinical procedure where the clinician helps the patient repeatedly visualize being exposed to a certain obsessive cue without ritualizing until that cue or situation no longer evokes anxiety or discomfort

satiation — a clinical procedure where the clinician has the patient verbalize ruminations while the clinician encourages the patient through the use of verbal prompts

aversion relief — the process of punishing behavior followed by the ending of the punishment when the person stopped thinking the undesired thoughts or displaying undesired behaviors

thought stopping — disrupting thoughts by having the person use the word or image, "Stop!" immediately following the thought to be prevented

These early behavioral treatments for OCD included some form of exposure to obsessive material. However, rituals were often not included in treatment, and this may be why most of these approaches proved only partially effective in OCD treatment. Currently, the far more successful behavioral treatment of exposure and response prevention incorporates the more helpful aspects of these early interventions, such as exposure to the feared stimuli.

Exposure and Response Prevention

Currently the most effective psychological treatment for OCD is *exposure and response prevention*. This therapy employs prolonged exposure to obsessional cues and prevention of compulsive rituals.[47] Exposure and response prevention consists of two main components, that is *in-vivo* or *imagined exposure* followed by *response prevention*.

In-vivo and/or imagined exposure elicit anxiety in the patient for periods of one to two hours. Then, the clinician asks the patient to refrain from performing any compulsions while anxiety levels decrease. Response prevention is always included in imagined exposure scenes and always follows exposure in-vivo. These treatment methods are described in step-by-step fashion by Steketee in the book, ***Treatment of Obsessive Compulsive Disorder,*** and summarized below.[32]

> ▶ **In-vivo exposure** — Exposure in-vivo consists of approximately one to two hours of actual confrontation with the feared stimulus; however, relaxation techniques are not utilized because they have not proven helpful and are unlikely to be useful when patients are experiencing high levels of anxiety or discomfort.[46] In initial consultations with the clinician, each patient determines a hierarchy of feared situations from low anxiety-producing situations to extreme anxiety-producing situations. Based on this hierarchy, anxiety-evoking objects or situations are introduced to the patient in a gradual or hierarchical manner, starting with items that evoke moderate discomfort. The clinician presents each object or situation in the hierarchy until the patient experiences significantly less anxiety or distress. At this point, treatment proceeds to the next exposure item on the hierarchy.
>
> With many obsessions, in-vivo exposure in the clinician's office is not feasible. For example, one could not replicate in an office a patient's obsessive thoughts that he or she just hit someone on the road with a car. However, a number of cleaning, checking, and counting obsessions are amenable to in-vivo exposure in the clinician's office. For an obsessive cleaner, a clinician might present

exposure and response prevention — the patient confronts obsessional cues and is prevented from performing compulsions

in-vivo exposure — exposure to the actual anxiety-eliciting stimulus, such as a garbage can

imagined exposure — exposure to the feared stimuli through the use of mental imagery

response prevention — deliberate blocking of overt and mental rituals and obsessive avoidance behaviors

small quantities of dirt or some other contaminant and ask the patient to run his or her hands through it and rub it on the face, hair, and clothes. For a compulsive counter, a clinician might require the patient to take 13 steps or perform some action involving an anxiety-provoking number.

A technique that may be useful during in-vivo exposure is *modeling*. In participant modeling, the clinician first demonstrates the desired behavior by making contact with the feared object, and then asks the patient to do the same. Modeling may also be passive: the clinician performs the target behavior while asking the patient to closely observe. Unlike participant modeling, the patient is not asked to perform the behaviors. Passive modeling may achieve some symptom reduction but is inferior to participant modeling.[48]

modeling — a technique where the clinician demonstrates exposure for the patient

▶ **Imagined exposure** — Imagined exposure is used whenever in-vivo exposure is impossible (e.g., with fear of a coworker dying of a heart attack or a son injured by a car). The clinician presents the patient with a series of scenes, (usually between four and 10), in increasing order of difficulty based on their hierarchical list of feared situations. This presentation starts with the least-feared scene and ends with the most-feared one. To induce the patient into each feared situation, the clinician describes the event, object, or situation, including many sensory details, until the patient has a clear picture of that stimulus context in mind. For example, with a compulsive checker, the clinician may describe a scene where the patient imagines he or she has failed to check the stove properly, and the house catches fire. The clinician describes the situation, the patient's actions, and the possible adverse consequences that the patient fears may arise from the failure to check.

The clinician presents each scene continuously or repeats it several times until the patient experiences considerably less anxiety or distress in response to that stimulus. The time required to complete a situation varies greatly between patients. Therapy sessions usually last between one and two hours, so it is sometimes necessary to use more than one session to complete one scene. At that point, the clinician presents the next scene in the hierarchy, continuing on until the patient can experience all scenes without increased anxiety or distress.

Imagined exposure differs from systematic desensitization in two ways:

1. Instead of being paired with relaxation, exposure scenes are intended to elicit at least moderate levels of anxiety from the patient. This anxiety shows habituation or reduction over time.

2. All scenes include response prevention so the patient does not imagine performing compulsions.

▶ **Response prevention** — Response prevention involves prohibiting the ritualistic behavior either during or between therapy sessions for prolonged periods of several hours to days. Response prevention is self-imposed by the patient; it is never enforced by the clinician or anyone else with the use of physical restraint. During the therapy session, the clinician explains the importance of response prevention and describes feelings the patient will likely experience. At home, a friend or relative often plays the role of the supporter, encouraging the patient during the self-imposed response prevention to the feared objects or situations. Response prevention is essentially the same regardless of the compulsion being prohibited. It simply involves the patient waiting for long periods after exposure to a feared situation, such as a garbage can, without performing any compulsive rituals like hand washing or showering to alleviate the anxiety. Compulsive urges gradually decline. Usually, the rituals are never permitted at all after exposure; although, in some cases, a brief ritual may be allowed if circumstances require.

Behavior therapy is something the patients have to do themselves. Thus, the clinician acts much like a training coach, designing workouts (homework assignments) that become progressively more difficult.

Most exposure and response prevention occurs outside of therapy sessions due to expense and time constraints. The combination of exposure and response prevention as a therapy program does not easily fit the typical, 50-minute therapy session. Some exposures can be accomplished in the clinician's office; however, most require the patient to self-administer the therapy with the help of a support person between scheduled therapy sessions. Patients can designate a friend or relative to be this support person, having them remind the patient of the rationale and instructions for using response prevention. Neither support persons nor clinicians may force the patients to do anything against their will.

Some research indicates that for people with milder cases of OCD, self-exposure and self-imposed ritual prevention are as effective as exposure and response prevention guided by a clinician.[49, 50] Additionally, computerized exposure treatment programs are currently under investigation for their utility in treating OCD.[51-56]

The process of response prevention differs for various patients, depending on their compulsive rituals. Long exposure periods have been found to be more effective than brief, interrupted exposures.[5] The exposure must not be terminated while the patient's distress or anxiety level remains high, usually at least 30 minutes. Therefore, exposure sessions should last at least 45 minutes.[5] The optimum frequency of exposure sessions has not been studied, but clinical observation suggests that frequent or daily sessions are preferable in severe cases, though two to three sessions per week may be sufficient in moderate cases. When self-exposure homework between treatment sessions can be assessed, the clinician may be able to use weekly sessions with periodic telephone contacts to check on homework progress.

> *The clinician requires the patient to keep accurate records of self-imposed response prevention to facilitate follow-up at the next session.*

Efficacy of Behavioral Treatment Approaches

Approximately 25 percent of those with OCD refuse to participate in behavior therapy. However, those who faithfully expose themselves and remain in contact with anxiety-evoking situations without performing rituals until their anxiety lessens have pronounced reductions of rituals and discomfort associated with their obsessions.[57] Of those who commit themselves to behavior therapy, less than 10 percent fail to complete it.

> *People who comply with behavioral treatments do so despite the induced anxiety because they believe the long-term benefits outweigh the short-term discomfort.*

Behavior therapy appears to be most indicated for those with OCD symptoms of:[58]

▶ Aggressive checking

▶ Contamination/cleaning

▶ Symmetry/ordering

Research reviewed in this section covers:

▶ Initial OCD behavioral treatments

▶ More effective treatments using exposure and response prevention

▶ Variations in exposure and response prevention, including presentation of stimuli in treatment, level of supervision for treatment, and the treatment of mental rituals

Initial OCD Behavioral Treatments

Early behavioral treatments, such as systematic desensitization, satiation, and paradoxical intention are not as effective in treating OCD as current methods. Initially, systematic desensitization was reported as rather effective. However, later case reports indicated that it reduced symptoms in only 30 to 40 percent of patients and often required many treatment sessions.[46, 59, 60] Systematic desensitization was found to be more effective when:

▶ Combined with in-vivo exposure; exposure to the actual feared stimuli produced change in 60 percent of patients.

▶ There was a recent onset of symptoms rather than when used with individuals experiencing chronic OCD.

However, the effectiveness of systematic desensitization is questionable because these findings are based on small numbers of case reports. *Controlled research studies* on larger populations are needed to establish systematic desensitization as a viable treatment alternative for OCD.

As a whole, paradoxical intention, satiation, aversion relief, and thought stopping are only partially successful in the treatment of OCD.[5]

Exposure and Response Prevention

Efficacy research indicates that exposure and response prevention is not indicated for individuals who:[5, 19, 58, 61]

▶ Are seriously depressed or delusional

▶ Undermine therapy with overt or covert rituals or avoidance techniques

▶ Present the symptom of hoarding (they tend to drop out of therapy)

▶ Have sexual/religious obsessions

▶ Are convinced that obsessive worries or repetitive behaviors are realistic or rational

Studies have shown that imagined exposure alone for OCD is an ineffective treatment. However, when combined with in-vivo exposure, imagined exposure helps maintain the gains achieved with in-vivo exposure.[32] *Meta-analyses* of exposure and response prevention controlled-outcome studies indicate that the combination of exposure and response prevention was highly successful in reducing obsessions and compulsions.[62–64] This treatment yielded at least a 70 percent reduction in obsessions and rituals in 51 percent of those who completed a course of treatment. In addition, 39 percent of the patients had a 30 to 69 percent reduction in obsessions and rituals. In other words, 90 percent of the individuals with OCD who complied with exposure and response prevention experienced moderate improvement, were much improved, or "recovered" by the end of treatment.

An additional published overview of OCD behavior therapy outcome studies confirmed that 80–90 percent of patients treated were classified as improved, with up to 80 percent reduction in

controlled research studies — research studies in which the various treatments in the study are regulated so that causal factors can be unambiguously identified

For those "treatment-refractory" patients, biological treatments (reviewed in the next chapter) and cognitive treatments (reviewed on pages 32–37 of this chapter) may enable them to respond better to behavior therapy.

meta-analysis — a study of the collective findings of many individual outcome studies to give an overall level of effectiveness for a certain type of treatment

symptom severity.[19] Even with dropouts and those who refuse treatment included, 63 percent of those with OCD achieved some symptom improvement from behavior therapy.[19]

Study results also indicate that approximately 70 to 80 percent of patients with OCD treated with this procedure remained improved at follow-up, though follow-up times varied among studies.[19, 48] Several factors, though controversial, have been linked with a positive treatment outcome. These factors include early onset of symptoms and lower levels of pretreatment anxiety and depressed mood. On the other hand, symptom duration was not found to correlate with treatment outcome.[19, 32] Other factors affecting this therapy include:

> ▶ **Level of supervision** — The clinician's supervision during exposure and response prevention appears insignificant for outcome effect.[5] Treatment is equally successful regardless of clinician involvement. Further, patients engaging in self-directed exposure and response prevention therapy following treatment guidelines in a book show modest improvement.[65] Although limited, research results appear to indicate self-imposed response prevention is just as effective as response prevention under 24-hour supervision.[49] Results achieved in studies with strict response prevention are somewhat mixed. In early studies, slightly better results occurred.[5, 32] However, Abramowitz et al. recently compared the effectiveness of intensive versus twice-weekly sessions of exposure and ritual prevention. Both programs were effective. At post-treatment, the intensive group appeared to have more improvement. Additionally, there was evidence of relapse in the intensive group but not in the twice-weekly group.[67]

> ▶ **Presentation of stimuli** — With most patients, it does not matter if anxiety-provoking stimuli are presented hierarchically, beginning with the least distressing, or whether the most distressing stimulus is presented at treatment outset.[68] However, clinical observations suggest that patients are more receptive to a treatment program that gradually approaches their most-feared situations.[5]

> ▶ **Mental rituals** — These are more difficult to treat than overt behavioral rituals because they are harder to identify and cannot be observed by the clinician. Therefore, behavioral treatment of individuals with mental rather than behavioral rituals has not been generally as successful. Patients who have mental compulsions have less control over their occurrence because, unlike active behaviors, there is little time or distinction between the urge to perform mental rituals and their actual performance.[5]

"The St. Louis Model," for treating patients with OCD who have treatment-interfering behaviors (TIBs) shows preliminary success, but needs more research. The model uses problem solving, family consultation, emotion-management strategies, and confronting incompatible treatment beliefs to deal with TIBs before a patient is allowed to continue behavior therapy or pharmacological treatment trials.[66]

The addition of cognitive therapy techniques to behavior therapy (that specifically targets mental rituals) appears to be very helpful in treating mental rituals.[69]

What is the Cognitive Therapy Approach to Treating OCD?

Cognitive theorists believe that people with OCD have an impaired ability to organize and integrate information. They may respond to and process emotional cues with greater difficulty and discomfort, and they may misinterpret intrusive thoughts so that these become obsessions. This section reviews:

▶ Cognitive theories related to OCD

▶ Cognitive treatment strategies

▶ Efficacy research for using Cognitive Therapy with OCD

One cognitive explanation of OCD suggests that individuals suffer from the disorder because they have unusually high expectations of negative outcomes (e.g., believing they will die from touching a garbage can). In addition, they overestimate the negative consequences for a variety of actions (e.g., believing they have hit someone with their car when they have simply hit a pot hole or driven over a bump in the road).[5] Obsessional content typically involves exaggerations of normal concerns (e.g., health, death, welfare of others, sex, and religion).

Cognitive theorists believe that people with OCD suffer from some common *irrational beliefs* associated with obsessive fears.[70] These beliefs include:

irrational beliefs — false perceptions of reality based on exaggerated expectations

▶ Having a thought about doing an action is the same as performing the action.

▶ Not trying to prevent harm to self or others is the same as having caused the harm in the first place.

▶ Being personally responsible for thoughts or actions remains unchanged by other factors, such as a low probability that an event may occur or that others have a role in event outcomes.

▶ Failing to correct or undo an aggressive or violent thought equates to seeking or wanting such harm to actually happen.

▶ Exercising control over one's thoughts is mandatory.

▶ Being especially vigilant prevents disasters.

▶ Being absolutely certain that no harm has or will occur is important.

▶ Not performing perfectly is the same as failing.

In a recent article, Libby et al. suggest that cognitive appraisals in children and adolescents with OCD are similar to those of adults with the disorder.[74]

Some cognitive theorists believe that normal intrusive thoughts may turn to obsessions when the person interprets or appraises the intrusion as potentially harmful and takes responsibility for causing this harm.[71-73] This appraisal leads to increased anxiety and guilt. The individual then develops avoidance behaviors and overt or covert compulsions to reduce the anxiety. The key element in this view of OCD is the negative automatic thoughts or interpretations that accompany intrusive experiences.[70] These thoughts may include, "Did I forget to check the stove and oven? I can't take the chance, or my house is going to burn down," or "Thinking about an accident makes me responsible for preventing it."

Another cognitive explanation for people with OCD is that they hold very basic erroneous beliefs, such as, "One must be completely competent in all endeavors to be worthwhile; therefore, I can't make any mistakes."[75] These erroneous beliefs lead to perfectionist striving that then provokes anxiety. Additionally, patients with OCD may believe they cannot tolerate the anxiety and therefore devalue their ability to adequately deal with such threats. This dysfunctional cycle continues when individuals with OCD doubt that they can cope with the possibility of negative outcomes. Cognitive theorists view compulsions, such as "I must turn the car around and check to be sure I did not hit someone," as attempts to reduce the overestimated harm and excessive sense of responsibility they feel.

OCD reflects an impairment, not in the content, but in the organization and integration of thinking.[21] OCD seems to involve memory deficits or at least a lack of confidence in memory. Those with OCD perceive information correctly; however, many have difficulties interpreting and making use of that information. Individuals with OCD repeatedly perform their compulsive rituals because they are not convinced that they have adequately processed information about threat.

For example, an individual will check the car lights again and again, forgetting or doubting that they were already checked. Similarly, a man may turn his car around repeatedly to check if he hit a person on the road because he mistrusts his experiences.

Cognitive Treatment Methods

Cognitive theories about the origin of OCD appear to fall between psychodynamic and behavioral explanations. This is because these theories focus on cognitions like thoughts or images that are internal to obsessive-compulsives but affect behaviors and patterns of reinforcement. Two main cognitive techniques have been used in OCD treatment:

1. Challenging of obsessional thoughts using Albert Ellis' rational emotive therapy (RET)[77]
2. Challenging negative automatic thoughts using Aaron Beck's cognitive therapy, which focuses on negative automatic rather than on only obsessional thoughts[78]

*Clark's **Cognitive-Behavioral Therapy for OCD** offers a good summary of cognitive research on OCD, which the author integrated into a "Cognitive Control Theory of Obsessions." The book also presents a cognitive treatment model (yet to be well researched) that addresses this theory.[76]*

Rational Emotive Therapy (RET)

The essential element of this treatment involves determining what types of generalized irrational thoughts and mistaken assumptions control the patient's negative feelings of anxiety, discomfort, and tension. The cognitive clinician then works to change the patient's irrational thoughts so that he or she no longer feels undue discomfort or anxiety. When the patient no longer feels discomfort, theorists believe that compulsions are no longer needed to reduce these negative feelings.

For example, with a compulsive cleaner, a clinician would first help the patient realize the irrationality of thoughts like, "If I touch a garbage can, I will become ill and maybe die," or "I must wash my hands many times before I am really clean." The clinician then works with the patient to revise the irrational thoughts and develop more accurate perceptions of threat, such as: "Touching garbage cans will not harm me," or "One wash is sufficient to clean my hands." Once the patient replaces irrational thoughts with more accurate ones, he or she will no longer perform compulsions because the threat and anxiety that prompted them are no longer present.

RET makes use of Ellis' ABC framework (see figure 3.1 on the next page) in which "Activating Events" (situational triggers) elicit "Beliefs" (rational and irrational), which are the direct source of emotional and behavioral "Consequences" (obsessions, compulsions, or discomfort).[75, 77] The focus of therapy works to modify these thoughts so that undue feelings of discomfort are no longer experienced. At that point, the compulsive rituals are no longer necessary.

Before therapy begins, the patient reads an explanation of RET written in simple terms.[79] Reading this helps the patient understand how to analyze irrational beliefs during homework assignments. Treatment begins with the clinician training the patient to observe and record cognitions, using pre-coded ABC homework sheets to help discriminate between the actual event and thoughts about the event. During the next therapy stage, the patient and clinician rationally dispute the irrational cognitions that the patient logged on the homework sheets. The clinician challenges the irrational beliefs using *Socratic questioning*, and the patient is instructed to do the same on homework assignments. For example, a patient may ask, "What are the chances of that horrible consequence actually occurring? What proof do I have of that being the best explanation?" The clinician requires the patient to practice analyzing problems with the pre-coded ABC homework sheets. When homework problems arise, the clinician discusses these with the patient, and they analyze the irrational beliefs associated with the problems.

Socratic questioning — posing a series of questions to force the patient to defend irrational beliefs, such as: "What evidence do you have to support that idea? What's the likelihood of such an outcome? What are other possible explanations?"

Figure 3.1   Rational Emotive Therapy (RET) Components

- **Activating Events** — Situational triggers, such as seeing a speed limit sign while driving

- **Beliefs** — Rational and irrational thoughts, such as "If I am not absolutely sure of the speed limit, I will cause an accident"

- **Consequences** — Obsessions and discomfort; for example, repeatedly going back and checking the speed limit sign

ACTIVATING EVENTS
(Situational Triggers)

▼

BELIEFS
(Rational and Irrational)

▼

CONSEQUENCES
(Depression, Anger, Suicide Attempts)

Beck's Cognitive Therapy

Unlike RET, Beck's cognitive therapy focuses on challenging negative automatic thoughts or interpretations associated with intrusions. These *negative automatic thoughts* differ from obsessional thoughts in that they are broader, more generalized, and pertain to the meaning patients attach to their obsessive thoughts. For example, a person's automatic thoughts may include: "I'm a dangerous person and may lose control at any moment," "I do not have the skills to cope with my problems," or "People would reject me if they knew about my thoughts." On the other hand, obsessional thoughts might be: "If I do not check the stove again, the house may burn down," or "If I do not wash my hands again, I will catch a disease." These negative interpretations of intrusive experiences are thought to be precursors of obsessional thoughts.[73, 79, 80]

> **negative automatic thoughts** — immediate interpretations about the meaning of obsessive thoughts

Challenging these automatic thoughts is similar to using RET. The clinician first identifies the themes contained in responses to intrusive experiences, using thought-recording forms that the patient completes for homework. The clinician then challenges the patient's thinking in a Socratic-like fashion with questions and restatements of the patient's reported beliefs. This dialogue forces the patient to defend and explain rationally his or her irrational thinking, helping the patient realize the unreasonable and detrimental nature of those thoughts. This begins a process of learning new, more adaptive reactions to intrusive, obsessional ideas. Specific cognitive therapy techniques have been developed to address patients' irrational beliefs about the over-importance and need to control thoughts, the probability of danger, and excessive responsibility.[73, 79]

Two of these techniques are called "Probability Estimation" and "Responsibility Pie":

► **Probability estimation** — In probability estimation, the clinician and patient identify events that would have to occur for the feared disaster to happen and then estimate the actual likelihood of each event. Multiplying these probabilities together usually gives the patient a clear idea of exactly how unlikely the feared disaster would be. Often, the probability can be expressed in the number of lifetimes the person with OCD would have to live to witness the event.

► **Responsibility pie** — To estimate responsibility, the clinician draws a pie and asks the patient to generate a list of all other persons or organizations that might play some role in the feared outcome (e.g., cooking food that might harm a guest). After assigning percentages of responsibility to each of these (e.g., food maker, storage facilities, transporters, distributors, sellers, etc.), usually very little responsibility is left to the preparer to cause harm.

Efficacy of Cognitive Treatment Approaches

Since obsessive compulsive symptoms are accompanied by and partly maintained by irrational cognitions, one would expect that cognitive therapy would be extremely popular and effective in treating OCD.[81] However, the limited research results from studies of cognitive therapy effectiveness to date have been inconclusive. For example:

► A recent study of 22 patients with OCD found cognitive therapy that reduced beliefs related to disease or contamination threat to be more effective than exposure and response prevention behavior therapy.[82]

► Several uncontrolled case studies have shown successful OCD treatment with cognitive therapy alone or in addition to exposure and response prevention.[21, 80]

► Other published controlled studies have found cognitive therapy for OCD to be effective, although not more so than exposure and response prevention alone.[69, 81, 83–85]

► Other research indicates that the combination of cognitive therapy and exposure and response prevention was no more effective than exposure and response prevention alone.[62, 83]

Some controlled studies indicate that both RET and Beck's cognitive therapy are effective for treating some patients with OCD. For example:

▶ **RET effectiveness** — Two controlled studies have been conducted comparing cognitive treatment (based on RET techniques) with exposure and response prevention and found no differences between the two treatments in either study. Both RET and self-controlled exposure and response prevention reduced obsessive-compulsive symptoms as well as social anxiety.[81, 83] Additionally, RET significantly reduced depression scores.[81] Thus, RET may be especially successful for people with OCD who are also depressed.

▶ **Beck's cognitive therapy effectiveness** — Two controlled studies of Beck's cognitive therapy focused on challenging negative automatic thoughts. Results indicate that this treatment was at least as good as exposure and response prevention in one trial, with nearly 75 percent of participants improved.[84] Further, an 84 percent success rate was achieved when cognitive therapy was combined with exposure and response prevention in patients who had obsessions and mental rituals but no overt compulsions.[69]

At present, insufficient information exists about whether patients with severe depression, *over-valued ideation*, or obsessions without behavioral rituals benefit more from cognitive therapy than from exposure and response prevention.[78] However, one must still be cautious about the effectiveness of cognitive therapy alone in the treatment of OCD. More research is needed to determine the best cognitive therapy techniques for OCD and which patients will benefit most from this method.

What is the Psychoanalytic Approach to Treating OCD?

Modern psychoanalytic approaches promote the concept that current psychological problems result from historical experiences and personality development. There is no research indicating that this approach is effective in treating OCD. However, psychoanalytic treatment focuses on understanding the disorder and resolving early traumatic experiences that may be related to OCD symptoms.

See pages 54–55 for an explanation of the brain areas and cognitive processes involved in the maintenance and treatment of OCD.

Since patients with obsessions and mental rituals, but no overt compulsions, have traditionally been very difficult to treat, the successful outcome from cognitive and behavioral treatments combined is quite remarkable.

over-valued ideation — belief that obsessive fears are realistic

Psychoanalytic Treatment Methods

In the past, psychoanalytic treatments often lasted many months or even years. In more recent years, changes in health care have led to the development of short-term psychoanalytic treatments for OCD, in which the clinician attempts to help patients face the sources of their anxiety and understand the ineffective compulsions they use to deal with these defense mechanisms.

The main components of psychoanalytic treatment are:

> **Providing** *insight* — Short-term, analytic treatment is very active and involves directly producing *insight* to the patient. The clinician achieves this by exposing the patient to underlying conflicts through *interpreting* how the patient's current statements and actions reflect underlying conflicts and wishes.

insight — self-awareness or self-understanding of the underlying dynamics of one's actions

interpreting — the clinician reflects to the patient hypotheses regarding the connection between unconscious material and current or conscious feelings or behavior

ego strength — self-confidence, resourcefulness, stability, and ability to cope with problems and stresses in life situations

> **Tolerating anxiety** — Because interpretations can produce great anxiety, patients must have the *ego strength* to withstand anxiety-provoking interpretations and insight.[86] Ego-strength characteristics include being motivated to change, possessing above-average psychological sophistication, and having had a meaningful relationship during childhood.

> **Psychoanalytic formulation of symptoms and defenses** — After taking the patient's personal history and making sure he or she meets selection criteria, (e.g., ego strength) for short-term psychoanalytic treatment, the clinician develops and communicates an analytic formulation that offers a resolution to the patient's problems. Together, clinician and patient reach an agreement on this view of the problem before proceeding.[86]

corrective emotional experience — when a patient reexperiences with the clinician an old, chronic conflicting pattern of behavior, such as extreme dependency, and the therapeutic relationship allows for a different healing outcome to the old pattern of behavior

positive transference — the patient recalls and relives pleasant experiences, feelings, and memories from the past as if they were occurring in the present

> **Corrective emotional experience in the therapy relationship** — By establishing a therapeutic alliance or bond between the clinician and the patient early in the therapeutic relationship, a *corrective emotional experience* often results that helps the patient solve conflicts. Using *positive transference*, the result can be a powerful motivating force, compelling the patient to give up maladaptive behaviors.[86]

> **Active confrontation** — The clinician directly confronts the patient with paradoxical behavior patterns and uses clear examples to clarify the connection between current difficulties and past experiences.

During the course of short-term psychodynamic treatment, the clinician continually encounters the patient's defense mechanisms. These defenses may involve:

> Denial of excessive compulsive rituals

> Resistance to discussing obsessions

> Rationalizing the compulsion as logical

Clarifying and resolving the patient's defenses throughout treatment helps patients to gain insight into early events in childhood that produce obsessive-compulsive symptoms and to continue moving toward treatment goals.

Efficacy of Psychoanalytic Treatment Approaches

Unfortunately, there are no adequate outcome research studies on psychoanalytic treatments for OCD. In fact, one appraisal concluded that cure of even uncomplicated cases by this approach is uncommon.[61] Although research fails to confirm psychoanalytic treatments as effective for OCD, this approach may help some patients work out early traumatic experiences that may be troubling to them in other spheres (e.g., social anxiety in the presence of others). Freed of OCD's debilitating symptoms, patients may be able to work on coexisting psychological issues of denial, avoidance, and dependency that may have been involved in the development and persistence of OCD.[87]

What is the Group Therapy Approach to Treating OCD?

In this era of managed care and health care reform, using group behavior psychotherapy to treat OCD can be cost-effective as well as therapeutically useful. First, group therapy is more cost-effective than individual OCD therapy because it requires far fewer staff hours to treat the same number of patients. Second, group OCD treatment increases the availability of therapy for areas with limited, trained behavior clinicians.[88] Third, therapeutic factors uniquely associated with group therapy may enhance the treatment efficacy of individual behavior therapy. These therapeutic factors include:

- ▶ **Universality** — The awareness that other patients suffer similar symptoms and the growing understanding that OCD is widespread, help to break down the patient's feelings of loneliness and isolation. This is especially helpful because those with OCD often isolate themselves due to the embarrassing nature of their symptoms. Sharing feelings and symptoms with others having similar problems helps to overcome the stigma, shame, and loneliness associated with the illness.[88]

- ▶ **Altruism** — In a group, patients with OCD come to realize that they have something to contribute to others in terms of suggestions, support, feedback, and reassurance.[88] By helping others, they begin to regain a sense of self worth.

▶ **Vicarious learning** — Members of an OCD treatment group can learn by observing others working through similar issues. Because patients listen to others engage in goal setting and behavioral treatments, group members teach and learn from each other as well as acting as motivating examples.

▶ **Interpersonal learning** — Patients with OCD often lose perspective as to what is normal behavior. Most group members suffer from different OCD symptoms. Therefore, several members in any group will behave quite normally in many areas of their lives that are problematic for other group members. Group members can learn from each other appropriate behavior for the "normal" person and set goals accordingly.[88]

▶ **Role flexibility** — Each member can act both as a patient and as a facilitator. Role flexibility enables group members to work as facilitators, coaches, and guides for one another.[88]

group cohesiveness — the degree to which group members work together for the benefit of each other and the group as a whole

▶ *Group cohesiveness* — Cohesive groups have a sense of trust, warmth, understanding, acceptance, and solidarity. Setting goals in the presence of the group is an important motivating factor because members are aware that they must share their progress with others at the next meeting. The group atmosphere often helps patients develop larger social support networks as well as spend less time ruminating.[89]

Group Therapy Treatment Methods

There are well-developed guidelines describing the logistics and screening procedures used to manage OCD groups.[89-92] Treatment methods discussed in this section focus on two similar yet distinct behavioral group therapy programs:

Individuals who complete group therapy may feel more comfortable joining community OCD support groups because the stigma and shame of the disorder have been removed.[89]

1. Methods used in a psychoeducational and support group for patients with OCD that can help those who are also receiving or have received individual behavior therapy or medication therapy

2. Methods used in group behavioral treatment that include in-vivo and imagined exposure as well as response prevention

Group behavioral therapy for OCD has some potential limitations, including:

► **Difficulty organizing a treatment group** — In some settings, the number of those suffering from OCD who seek treatment may not be adequate to form a group. At least six patients are needed to begin a group.[88]

► **Fearing that new symptoms will be acquired** — Although some patients fear acquiring new OCD symptoms, studies on behavioral group therapy for OCD show this very rarely happens.[88] If it does occur, the group leader can refer the patient to individual therapy.

► **Noncompliance with treatment** — When noncompliance occurs because of a homework problem, the clinician can use discussion and problem solving to determine a homework task with which the patient will comply.

► **Missed therapy sessions** — Patients may avoid coming to the group if they failed to do homework tasks. In this case, the group leader can give these patients homework tasks at a more appropriate difficulty level.

Psychoeducational Group Therapy

Psychoeducational support groups help clarify the nature of OCD and available treatments. They are intended to facilitate concurrent treatment or to help patients and their families decide on what treatment they would like.

A typical psychoeducational and support group may meet once a week for 10 weeks to educate patients and families about OCD and to provide a support network.[90, 91] The outline can follow that of a self-help book for those with OCD, such as "When Once Is Not Enough," "Getting Control," or "Stop Obsessing."[93–95] Each session includes an informal lecture topic covered in the session's first 45 minutes. The final 30 to 45 minutes of the session is left open for questions and discussion of the topic covered.

The following lists each session's objectives:

► **Session 1** — Facilitator presents the group's purpose and goals as well as an overview of OCD symptoms and prevalence data.

► **Session 2** — Facilitator reviews OCD diagnostic criteria with relevant examples similar to symptoms found among group members as well as information about the relationship between OCD and other mental disorders.

► **Session 3** — Facilitator leads a discussion of what causes OCD and why it persists, often enhanced by a discussion of OCD-associated cognitions (e.g., irrational beliefs and inaccurate risk assessment).

Chapter four discusses the biological basis of OCD.

▶ **Session 4** — Group members receive instruction on OCD's biological basis, including information on the serotonin hypothesis and brain structures linked to OCD, followed possibly by a review of the research on the efficacy of medication treatment.

▶ **Session 5** — Facilitator gives an overview of OCD behavior therapy, covering exposure and response prevention. The group leader teaches patients to rate and rank their obsessions and compulsions on the Subjective Units of Distress (SUDs) scale. Each patient identifies approximately 10 situations, events, or objects that cause anxiety and ranks each according to how much anxiety it provokes. The facilitator may demonstrate gradual in-vivo exposure, using this to illustrate the effectiveness of individual OCD behavior therapy.

▶ **Session 6** — Participants receive information about exposure and response prevention and encouragement for group members to try relatively simple exposure and response prevention tasks during the session. For instance, an individual who fears being contaminated by touching another person may be asked to shake hands with one of the leaders or another group member without washing immediately afterward.

▶ **Session 7** — The group discusses the family's role in accommodating OCD and helping during treatment. Because family members can both help and hinder behavioral treatment's effectiveness, the group leader spends time explaining how the family members should and should not behave around the patient, especially during behavioral treatment.

Chapter four addresses pharmacotherapy for OCD.

▶ **Session 8** — Facilitator discusses current medications available for treating OCD as well as the side effects and limitations of pharmacotherapy, (e.g., augmenting agents occasionally used to treat OCD).

▶ **Session 9** — Facilitator discusses factors that promote successful treatment such as active involvement of the patient and family regardless of the treatment form used. At the end of the session, the group leaders discuss relapse prevention and the fact that OCD is a chronic disorder that may never completely subside.

▶ **Session 10** — The facilitator summarizes the previous sessions, discusses future directions for OCD research, and reviews group members' plans and involvement in current therapies.

Behavioral Treatment Group Therapy

Applying exposure and response prevention in a group setting requires identifying patients most likely to successfully respond in such a setting. Clinicians should follow these five steps before starting the group:[89, 92]

1. **Conduct a diagnostic assessment** — This involves making sure of an accurate diagnosis of OCD and possible coexisting conditions. Patients with schizophrenia and severe depression may manifest OCD-like symptoms, yet they would not respond well to group behavior therapy.

2. **Assess symptom type and severity** — By quantifying the degree of subjective distress caused by OCD symptoms, clinician and patient measure improvement during and after treatment. Individuals with a score above 30 on the Yale-Brown Obsessive-Compulsive Scale (see appendix A for a review of the Y-BOCS), are often not good group candidates because their daily functioning is too severely disabled. Individual treatment or pharmacotherapy may better serve these patients until their symptoms are more manageable.

3. **Recommend psychoeducational group therapy sessions** — Discussion of group composition and process helps patients make a smooth transition into the intensive and interactive behavioral treatment group sessions that will follow.

4. **Discuss treatment options** — The group leader and patient should discuss treatment options, getting a firm understanding of exposure and response prevention, without which the patient may be too frightened to enter such a treatment program. In such cases, the clinician discusses with the patient other treatment options including individual therapy or pharmacotherapy. Fearful patients may choose to join a group after engaging in other therapy.

5. **Develop a hierarchy of anxiety-evoking stimuli** — This is the final step before intensive, group behavioral treatment begins. A treatment staff member completes this task individually with each patient. The clinician and patient use the Subjective Units of Distress (SUDs) Scale (see page 14 in chapter two for a description of SUDs scales), to create a list of approximately 25 items or situations that cause anxiety to differing degrees. The clinician and patient order the items from least threatening to most threatening based on the scores assigned to each situation. This hierarchy is then ready for use during the group treatment.

There are two major phases of group behavior treatment: the intensive treatment phase and the maintenance treatment phase.

Intensive Treatment Phase

The group leader conducts two-hour sessions once or twice weekly over a period of up to 12 weeks with groups of six to 10 patients. During these sessions, patients are exposed to at least one situation listed on each person's hierarchy and are prevented from engaging in rituals. For example, an individual who fears being contaminated by a garbage can would be asked to touch a garbage can and then refrain from washing or cleaning rituals. An individual who fears the number 13 may be asked to take 13 steps and then refrain from undoing this.

For those obsessions impossible to introduce using in-vivo exposure during the group session, the patient is asked to imagine that situation as vividly as possible. For example, a compulsive checker would be asked to imagine leaving the house without checking any of the door locks, stove, or oven.

To achieve this with the best possible results, the clinician and patient construct a detailed script during an individual session that will be imagined during the group therapy session. To accommodate other group members' needs, scripts are generalized across different members' obsessive fears, while each patient pictures his or her own specific scenario.

In the last 30 minutes of the group session, the clinician focuses on assigning each patient homework tasks similar to the exposure and response prevention tasks described above. An individual who fears hitting people with a car would be assigned to drive around until those obsessions arose and then refrain from turning the car around and checking the road for injured pedestrians. The patient, clinician, and other group members take part in assigning exposure and response prevention tasks.

The first 30 minutes of each subsequent session generally consist of discussing the patients' experiences with the homework tasks. Those patients who were successful in their homework assignments are assigned the next situation or scene from their hierarchy until the most feared item in each patient's hierarchy is introduced.

In the final sessions, the clinician presents the patient with several situations simultaneously. This may be done in-vivo or in imagination. An example of a multiple in-vivo exposure and response prevention task may include a patient being asked to shake a person's hand, touch a trash can, pick up something from the bathroom floor, and touch the lavatory door handle, all without cleaning. A multiple, imagined exposure and response prevention task may include asking an individual to imagine:

▶ Not checking the car at night to make sure it hasn't been stolen

▶ Parking the car without checking the door locks, parking brake, and trunk

▶ Leaving the house without checking to make sure the iron, oven, stove, and curling iron are off

The specific tasks that individuals perform or imagine depend on their particular obsessions and compulsions. The exposure tasks for group treatment are very similar to those presented during individual exposure and response prevention.

Maintenance Treatment Phase

After the intensive therapy phase, patients often meet in behavior group therapy sessions spaced out gradually over the next few months.[89–92] These extra sessions motivate and support patients as they continue with exposure activities on their own. Group leaders also encourage patients to join local OCD support groups, if available.

Efficacy of Group Therapy

Group therapy is becoming a more common OCD treatment, either as a replacement for or adjunct to individual behavior therapy. Early uncontrolled studies of OCD behavioral group therapy indicate that group exposure and response prevention techniques effectively reduce OCD symptom severity in about 75 percent of participants.[92,96,97] Controlled studies from the 1990s that utilized detailed screening criteria and step-by-step procedures found behavioral group therapy as effective as individual behavior therapy at treatment completion as well as at a six-month follow-up.[89, 98] The only difference between the two treatments was that individual behavior therapy improved symptoms more quickly than group behavioral treatment.[98] Similarly, a more recent, uncontrolled study indicated that seven weeks of group exposure and response prevention therapy reduces obsessions, compulsions, and depression. Improvements were maintained at three- and six-month follow-up.[99] Another study recently found that cognitive-behavioral group therapy effectively reduced OCD symptom intensity and quicky improved patient quality of life, whether or not the patient was also taking medications for OCD.[100]

What is the Family Therapy Approach to Treating OCD?

Clinicians often recommend marital and family therapy as an adjunctive treatment for OCD, especially when the patient indicates that there are significant communication problems or conflicts at home. When the patient is married or lives with family, this therapy can be helpful in facilitating treatment gains as well as preventing relapse. Spouses and family members benefit greatly from being involved with the treatment and learning more about the disorder and how to cope with it. They begin to understand that it is not their fault that a family member suffers from OCD. They also learn effective means of coping instead of reinforcing or exacerbating the symptoms. Most importantly, learning about OCD lessens the stigma and shame associated with "mental disorders," which helps families to function more responsibly.[17, 33]

The family's role in successful OCD treatment is twofold:

1. They should be supportive towards the individual with OCD rather than angry or impatient. Hostile family reactions are especially discouraging to those with OCD and may lead to treatment dropout or failure.[101] However, family members should clearly express their concerns about OCD symptoms and encourage or even insist that their relative seek treatment.

2. Family members should refrain from overly accommodating and reinforcing the individual's obsessions or compulsions. Family members often reinforce the disorder unknowingly because they hate to see a loved one suffer through exhausting, compulsive rituals. In trying to help, family members may facilitate OCD symptoms and even perform the compulsions with and for the patient.[33] Although these behaviors may temporarily help reduce the patient's anxiety, they can exacerbate the disorder and its symptoms by reinforcing the obsessions and compulsions as rational and necessary. In addition, over-involved family members may inadvertently discourage treatment completion.[34]

Family Therapy Treatment Methods

Family members may be helpful assistants during the behavior therapy process. The most helpful family members will be adults (including spouses, partners, parents, or other relatives), whom the patient considers to be supportive and not overly intrusive in the patient's life.

Several components of family treatment are often employed.[35, 92] These include:

▶ **Family education** — Family members who will be assisting during treatment should attend some early sessions of the patient's therapy to learn more about OCD symptoms, etiology, and treatment methods. Educational sessions could be held individually with the patient or in a group setting with other OCD families.

▶ **Support training during exposure and response prevention** — Family assistants will need to learn to be helpful when the patient practices exposure and response prevention homework. The clinician can recommend what to say and do during exposure homework. For example, the clinician may recommend that the relative no longer reassure the patient. Instead, the family member may say, "I'm sorry, but Dr. Owen told me not to reassure you about your fears of hurting other people."

▶ **Reduced family accommodation** — In addition to supporting patients when they expose themselves to feared situations, family members will need to reduce their accommodation to the patient's OCD symptoms. This usually means not doing tasks for the patient and not performing rituals or checking at the patient's request. For example, the clinician may advise a family member not to take out the trash, wash hands, or check the stove, even if the patient requests it. These changes should be agreed upon together by the patient, the clinician, and the family member.

> *Family accommodation to their relative's OCD symptoms should be deliberately reduced during behavioral treatment.*

▶ **Communication and problem-solving training** — In some families, the patient and a family member have learned to communicate in angry ways or fail to discuss family problems related to OCD. When this happens, the clinician may ask the patient and family member to discuss OCD-related problems during the session. In this way, the clinician can stop ineffective, angry interchanges and encourage clear communication and problem solving. For example, the clinician might stop the relative from yelling at the patient about using the bathroom too much and ask what he or she would like to ask the patient to do instead. The clinician could then help negotiate a solution, such as reducing time in the bathroom, as part of the patient's exposure and response prevention homework.

Efficacy of Family Therapy Approaches

At the present time, only a few studies have investigated the benefits of family therapy. Several case reports have indicated that involving spouses or parents in behavioral treatment is very useful.[33] Surprisingly, two controlled studies have shown that including spouses as assistants during exposure and response prevention did not improve the patients' outcomes any more than uninvolved spouses. However, in a different study of family members in India, patients who were assisted by various types of relatives had more benefit than patients who were not helped by relatives.[33]

Recently, a small, pilot study suggested that cognitive-behavioral family therapy may be effective for children with OCD.[102] Subsequent research results indicate that both individual and group cognitive-behavioral, family-based therapy are equally effective in reducing OCD symptoms. Also, treatment gains were maintained at six-month follow up.[103]

Researchers have also studied multiple family treatment. When several family members participated together as a group with patients in behavioral treatment, patients showed considerable improvement in OCD symptoms.[92] Thus, it seems that including relatives in the behavioral treatment process can be very helpful.

Behavioral treatments are very successful in helping people with OCD. Using these treatments in a group setting or including family members may enhance the overall treatment program for some patients. However, many people (25 percent or more) are uncomfortable participating in behavior therapy and find relief from their symptoms through the use of medications. Other patients may respond well to the use of medications in combination with behavior therapy. The next chapter reviews how medications work in reducing OCD symptoms, commonly prescribed medications, and the research comparing the effectiveness of medication treatment versus behavioral treatment for OCD.

Key Concepts for Chapter Three:

1. The specific cause of OCD is unknown, but it is clear that biological, psychological, and environmental factors are involved.

2. The leading psychological treatments reflect behavioral and cognitive approaches.

3. The most effective psychological treatment for OCD is exposure and response prevention, in which the clinician exposes the patient to a feared stimulus and then prevents the patient from engaging in compulsive behaviors. As a result, anxiety levels gradually decrease.

4. Cognitive theorists attribute OCD to common irrational beliefs associated with obsessive fears. They work to change the patient's irrational thoughts so that the patient will no longer need to use compulsive behaviors to alleviate the fears that accompany those thoughts.

5. Cognitive therapy has been shown to be effective, but not as effective as exposure and response prevention.

6. Group therapy is becoming more popular as a treatment method, partly because it is less expensive. Early uncontrolled studies indicate effectiveness for group exposure and response prevention techniques.

Chapter 4:
Medical Treatment for Obsessive Compulsive Disorder

This chapter answers the following:

▸ **What is the Role of Genetics in the Development of Obsessive Compulsive Disorder (OCD)?** — This section reviews evidence for genetic underpinnings of OCD.

▸ **How are Brain Structures and Chemicals Related to OCD?** — This section reviews relevant research on neurobiological factors related to OCD.

▸ **What are the First-Line Medications Used to Treat OCD?** — This section reviews SRI medications used in OCD treatment, common side effects, efficacy research, and augmentation strategies.

▸ **What Other Medications are Used to Treat OCD?** — This section summarizes alternative medications that may prove useful in the treatment of OCD, especially for those who fail to respond to standard medication therapies.

▸ **What Other Biologically Based Treatments are Available for OCD?** — This section reviews unconventional but promising treatment strategies for patients with OCD who fail to respond to standard treatment regimens. These biological treatments include neurosurgery, electroconvulsive therapy, transcranial magnetic stimulation, and deep brain stimulation.

▸ **How Effective are Medications vs. Behavior Therapy for Treating OCD?** — This section reviews the comparative efficacy of the two primary treatment modalities for OCD.

ENVIRONMENTAL and psychological factors, such as childhood trauma, personality disturbances, and primitive coping skills have been historically implicated in the development of OCD. Over the past 25 years, however, a dramatic shift has occurred — now researchers widely acknowledge genetic and neurobiological factors as paramount in the development of the disorder.

What is the Role of Genetics in the Development of OCD?

Genetics has recently become one of the most active areas of OCD research. Although no specific gene(s) have been consistently associated with the disorder, there remains considerable evidence that genetic factors will eventually be identified as the key mediators of at least some specific OCD symptoms.

Authors of a recent OCD genetics literature review concluded that the disorder should be re-conceptualized as a heterogeneous illness comprised of several related, yet distinct sub-groups. By separating OCD into more homogeneous subgroups, the chance of identifying heritable components may well be enhanced.[104] They suggest an "OCD spectrum of related disorders that share some of the same vulnerability genes."[104] For example, there is considerable evidence supporting a genetic link between Tourette's syndrome and OCD symptoms, especially symmetry and ordering compulsions.

Additional research supports a link between the presence of certain symptom constellations and treatment response. For example, several groups have identified four primary symptom dimensions in OCD:

> ► Symmetry/ordering
>
> ► Hoarding (the best supported empirically)
>
> ► Contamination/cleaning
>
> ► Obsessions/checking

Mataiz-Cols et. al. reported that these primary symptom dimensions were associated with distinct characteristics related to comorbidity patterns, genetic transmission, neural substrates, and treatment response. Another recent review also concluded that there is considerable evidence that familial psychiatric disorders arise from genetically based biological traits or markers.[105] For example, decreased blood levels of serotonin and reduced serotonin receptor sensitivity may indicate a biological trait/marker for obsessions and compulsions.

Genetic (rather than environmental) factors appear to be paramount in accounting for the tendency of OCD to co-occur in families. Because a wide variance in individual symptom presentations often exists among family members, it is unlikely that familial links result from learned behavior. Other findings supporting the importance of genetic factors in OCD include:

> ► Those with OCD are more likely to have parents and children with the disorder and obsessive-compulsive behaviors than those who don't have OCD.[106–109]
>
> ► Approximately 40 percent of those with OCD also have a biological relative with OCD.[110]
>
> ► *Monozygotic* (identical) twins are more likely to exhibit OCD symptoms than *dizygotic* (fraternal/non-identical) twins.[107, 110]
>
> ► Results from family and twin studies indicate that a few, rather than multiple *genes*, are more likely to be critical in OCD development.[110]

monozygotic — derived from the same fertilized egg and identical genetic make-up

dizygotic — fraternal or non-identical twin derived from separate eggs and possessing different genetic characteristics

gene — DNA sequence located at a specific site on a chromosome that codes for a certain characteristic(s); the biological basis of heredity

Family studies provide further evidence for a genetic basis for OCD, suggesting that individuals with OCD are more likely to have biological relatives with other anxiety disorders and depression. This finding suggests that these disorders may share a similar underlying genetic basis as OCD. In fact, it is the prominent anxiety and frequent avoidance behaviors characteristic of OCD that support its current classification as an anxiety disorder. In addition, OCD is frequently complicated by the presence of comorbid depression and/or other anxiety disorders. Among individuals with OCD:

▶ Two-thirds will develop depression during their lifetime.[111-114]

▶ Ten percent will also meet criteria for bipolar disorder (manic-depressive) illness.[112, 113, 115]

▶ Forty percent will meet criteria for an additional anxiety diagnosis during their lifetime, especially: social phobia, panic disorder, or generalized anxiety disorder.[111-113]

> *Most studies have reported that panic disorder (10–35 percent), social phobia (10–40 percent), and generalized anxiety disorder (5–40 percent) are the most common co-existing anxiety disorders among those with OCD.[111-113]*

There is extensive evidence linking OCD and the neurological condition, Tourette's syndrome (TS).[116, 117] Most people with TS can voluntarily suppress their tics for short periods of time; however, tic suppression results in progressively worsening discomfort, so the tics eventually re-emerge. Research supporting a *genetic link* between OCD and TS indicates that:

▶ Over 50 percent of TS sufferers also experience OCD symptoms.[106]

▶ Individuals with OCD are four times more likely than those without OCD to have a family member with tics or TS.[107, 108, 110, 118]

▶ *Basal ganglia* dysfunction is implicated in both TS and OCD.[119, 120] (Same or similar genes may "code" vulnerability for TS and OCD.)[110]

genetic link — tendency for genes to be inherited together despite coding for separate characteristics and being located on different chromosome locations

basal ganglia — brain area comprised of several structures (including the caudate nucleus, putamen, and substantia nigra) that has a primary function to initiate and control body movements

How are Brain Structures and Chemicals Related to OCD?

Since the 1980s, researchers have demonstrated consistent neurobiological abnormalities as characteristic of OCD, including both neurochemical abnormalities and important differences in brain function, especially in specific brain regions. The behavioral effects elicited by certain brain injuries have also provided important clues about the specific sites within the brain most likely to mediate OCD symptoms.

Additional clues to the potential brain areas involved in OCD have come from:

> ▶ Studying the biological causes of other illnesses that produce OCD-like symptoms
>
> ▶ Conducting neuroimaging studies to examine structural and functional differences between individuals with OCD and those without OCD
>
> ▶ Investigating the underlying brain neuroanatomy
>
> ▶ Studying biochemical factors

Specific Brain Areas Involved

Numerous research investigations have demonstrated that OCD is characterized by abnormal hyperactivity in specific brain areas, notably within the orbital cortex, basal ganglia and *amygdala* (part of the *limbic system*), and *thalamus*.[121]

Basal Ganglia and Amygdala

Significant evidence implicates the **basal ganglia** in OCD symptom production based on its functional and structural characteristics:

The primary function of the basal ganglia is to transmit and modulate nerve impulses responsible for initiating and controlling movements.[23–25, 122–126] Additional functions of the basal ganglia include processing and filtering information about behaviors and cognitions that are being transmitted back to the basal ganglia from other brain regions (via the thalamus). Therefore, it is logical to conclude that the basal ganglia is likely to be the anatomical source for the development of symptoms related to abnormal behaviors (e.g., rituals).

In addition, a particularly rich array of *neurotransmitters* and multiple *receptors* are located at the site of the basal ganglia. Therefore, any disturbances occurring within the basal ganglia are likely to result in far-reaching consequences throughout the brain.

Research findings that suggest a link between **basal ganglia** damage/dysfunction and OCD symptoms include:

> ▶ In animal models, damage to the basal ganglia results in repetitive behaviors that resemble compulsive rituals.[28, 29, 125, 127–129]
>
> ▶ Tics and Tourette's syndrome are linked to basal ganglia dysregulation, especially hyperexcitability. OCD is also characterized by increased excitability in basal ganglia pathways, even in the absence of tics or Tourette's syndrome.[130]

amygdala — one of the basal ganglia that is part of the limbic system and believed to be involved in impulsivity and other functions

limbic system — brain region involved in smell, automatic behaviors, and emotions that surrounds the midbrain and has extensive connections with the thalamus and brain stem

thalamus — brain area with multiple connections to other brain regions that primarily functions as a relay station for body sensations, including pain and temperature

neurotransmitters — chemical messengers that transmit signals from one nerve cell to another to elicit physiological responses

receptors — membrane-bound protein molecules with highly specific shapes that function as "landing" sites for specific chemical messengers (neurotransmitters or medications)

▶ Patients afflicted with diseases involving basal ganglia deterioration (such as Parkinson's disease or Huntington's chorea) have an increased risk of subsequently developing OCD symptoms.[24, 131]

Findings from neuroimaging studies of patients with OCD that support the importance of the **amygdala** include:

▶ Increased activity in the amygdala when exposed to pictures of contaminated environments[132]

▶ Altered responses in the amygdala in comparison to control subjects when exposed to fearful as well as to neutral stimuli[133]

Pre-frontal and Orbito-frontal Brain Regions

Evidence implicating frontal lobe involvement in OCD relies on frontal-lobe–identified functions and results from neuroimaging studies (reviewed on pages 56–59).

The frontal lobes of the brain include pre-frontal and orbito-frontal regions. The primary functions mediated by the frontal lobes include:[23–25, 122–126]

▶ Filtering, prioritizing, and organizing information transmitted to the brain

▶ Suppressing or delaying responses triggered by extraneous or inconsequential stimuli

▶ Applying logical, prioritized, and consequence-based principles to interpret and respond to information as it is received

▶ Regulating and "fine-tuning" movements and complex behaviors activated by the basal ganglia

These functions are critical for filtering out extraneous thoughts and inhibiting responses to irrelevant internal as well as external stimuli.

Other Illnesses that Produce OCD-like Symptoms

Other illnesses or conditions that damage the basal ganglia and its connections to the brain's frontal lobes can elicit OCD-like symptoms (e.g., encephalitis, anoxia, and carbon-monoxide poisoning). Research on two disorders — Sydenham's chorea and pediatric autoimmune neuropsychiatric disorders associated with streptococcal infections (PANDAS) — further supports the importance of the basal ganglia in producing OCD symptoms.

See pages 10–11 and 16 for more complete lists of medical conditions associated with OCD symptoms.

Sydenham's chorea is a rare neurological condition that results when *antibodies* produced to combat group A, beta-hemolytic streptococcus bacteria in the brain mistakenly destroy basal ganglia nerve cells. Sydenham's chorea is characterized by rapid,

antibodies — complex protein molecules created specifically to destroy organisms deemed to be dangerous

purposeless, nonrepetitive movements of the extremities and is found in up to 10 percent of rheumatic fever cases.[134] Recent studies identify a link between Sydenham's chorea and OCD, supporting the role of the basal ganglia in producing OCD symptoms and indicating an elevated risk for individuals with Sydenham's chorea to subsequently develop OCD symptoms.[26, 135-137]

PANDAS is a term used to describe children with OCD whose OCD symptoms worsen after streptococcal infections. Current research indicates that PANDAS may result from an autoimmune-mediated inflammation of the basal ganglia.[138] Specifically, these researchers have found that:

> ▶ PANDAS is associated with group A, b-hemolytic streptococcal throat infections and responds favorably to appropriate antibiotic therapy.[139]

> ▶ The mechanism that underlies PANDAS can be linked with that of Sydenham's chorea.[140]

> ▶ The basal ganglia have a role in PANDAS (determined by comparing the MRIs (magnetic resonance imaging tests) of children with OCD who have had streptococcal infections to those of healthy children). Results indicate that the former have enlarged basal ganglia compared to counterparts who do not have OCD.[141]

> ▶ Higher antistreptococcal *antibody titers* that appear in patients with OCD are associated with structural alterations in the basal ganglia nuclei.[142]

A PANDAS diagnosis requires the presence of OCD and/or tic disorder; symptom onset between age three and puberty; an intermittent course of the disorder characterized by the onset of symptoms or by dramatic symptom exacerbations; symptom exacerbations associated with a streptococcal infection; and neurological abnormalities (tics, motoric hyperactivity).[33, 143, 144]

Neuroimaging Studies in OCD

Brain imaging studies use x-rays, *CAT (Computer Axial Tomography) scans*, and MRI examinations to evaluate brain structure and also brain function. In general, studies that have investigated brain structure in OCD have often identified subtle differences in brain structure in subjects with OCD versus those without OCD. However, no specific or unique abnormality in brain structure has been consistently identified that differentiates between those with and without OCD. Additionally, there is some evidence that people with OCD may have abnormal proportions when comparing one brain area to another. Although these findings are inconsistent and not particularly impressive, they suggest that structural brain abnormalities may not be uncommon in OCD.[23, 119, 122, 145-148]

One difference between Sydenham's chorea and PANDAS is that in PANDAS, OCD symptoms are present prior to a streptococcal infection and then exacerbated by the infection.

antibody titer — the dilution of a serum containing a specific antibody at which the solution just retains a specific activity (as neutralizing or precipitating an antigen), which it loses at any greater dilution

CAT (Computer Axial Tomography) scans — computer-assisted x-rays

Clearer and more compelling evidence of brain abnormalities exists from studies conducted to investigate brain function in OCD, including studies utilizing *PET, SPECT,* and MRI scans. Although these types of tests are not diagnostic (i.e., they can neither "make" nor "break" a specific diagnosis), they provide the following strong evidence that OCD is characterized by abnormal brain function:

PET — Positron Emission Tomography

SPECT — Single Photon Emission Computerized Tomography

▶ Most subjects with OCD have increased brain activity in the orbital-frontal region of the cerebral cortex compared to healthy volunteer subjects.[23, 119, 145, 146, 149]

▶ Some people with OCD have increased brain activity in the *caudate nucleus* within the basal ganglia of the brain compared to healthy volunteer subjects.[23, 119, 145, 146, 149]

caudate nucleus — a basal ganglia component involved in the voluntary control of movement

▶ Provoking OCD symptoms by exposing those with OCD to their most-feared stimuli results in increased activation of the orbital-frontal cortex and the basal ganglia on PET and SPECT scans of the brain.[23, 25, 146, 150]

▶ Patients with OCD that demonstrate hyperactivity in their frontal lobe or basal ganglia will have "normalized" brain activity when re-scanned only if successfully treated with an SRI antidepressant or behavior therapy.[44]

These neuroimaging studies have important and wide-ranging implications. Results suggest that certain brain abnormalities (excess activity in the frontal lobes and basal ganglia) are visible and measurable in most subjects with OCD. These brain abnormalities are considered *state like* rather than *trait like*. That is, inducing OCD symptoms elicits activation of the frontal lobes and the basal ganglia in subjects with OCD, and successful treatment results in "normalization" of the activity in these regions. Moreover, these changes in brain activity can

state like — circumstance-dependent characteristic

trait like — permanent, inherent characteristic

From The Patient's Perspective

Have seen Owen three times now. Jim's been great; thank God for his help. The pills seem to help relieve the worry some, and I'm more in control. I need to ask Owen about my sleep problems. I wonder if these are because of the medication. I'm starting to feel better — finally! I didn't have to repeat walking steps at all today. I still have bad times, especially when the baby is cranky and I'm tired. But, I finally feel like I am going to get this under control.

be detected whether or not improvement results from medication or behavioral interventions. Although behavioral therapy has traditionally been considered a non-biological treatment, successful OCD treatment with behavioral therapy appears to trigger chemical changes within the brain identical to those observed with successful medication treatment.[44]

Substantial evidence indicates that certain areas of the brain, specifically the frontal cortex, basal ganglia, and limbic system, are critical in the production of OCD symptoms (see figure 4.1 below). Specifically, neuroimaging studies indicate disturbance in the neural pathways that originate in the orbito-frontal cortex and traverse through the sub-cortical areas of the brain to terminate in the basal ganglia.

**Figure 4.1   Critical Brain Areas
Related to OCD Symptoms**

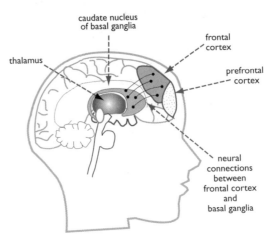

Some research indicates that input from the emotional (limbic) brain to the areas involved with cognitions (cortex) increases in comparison to the information flow from the frontal cortex back to the brain's limbic area. Therefore, the therapeutic effects attained with behavior therapy and medication treatments may be mediated at least in part by their ability to increase feedback in the weaker connections, resulting in a more normal flow of information between the limbic and cortical areas.

The circuit from the orbito-frontal to the sub-cortical parts of the brain is also critical in the production of OCD symptoms. Information received by the caudate nucleus of the basal ganglia is filtered and then transmitted to the orbito-frontal cortex for further interpretation and potential activation of appropriate responses. When this circuit is functioning properly, the portion originating in the basal ganglia and projecting to the cerebral cortex has an inhibitory effect. That is, increasing activity within the orbito-frontal to basal-ganglia pathway should trigger feedback from the returning portion of the loop. The resulting feedback suppresses further activation, preventing excess or superfluous behaviors.[150]

Several authors have postulated that inadequate filtering of anxiety-related inputs by the caudate nucleus could trigger the orbito-frontal cortex to initiate excessive behaviors, such as rituals. Impairment in the feedback mechanism could also encourage excess activation of behaviors or reduced ability to suppress behaviors once they occur. Evidence supporting this model includes:

▶ Patients with damage to the orbito-frontal circuit demonstrate an impaired ability to suppress their responses to irrelevant stimuli.[23, 123, 146]

▶ Subjects with OCD also demonstrate abnormal results in their ability to suppress inappropriate responses (suppression failure).[29, 123, 146, 151, 152]

▶ Abnormal activity in the basal ganglia occurs in subjects with OCD when they fail to suppress on tests administered during SPECT scans.[23]

Biochemical Factors in OCD

Most theories concerning OCD's etiology include some type of abnormal function in the neural circuits between the frontal lobe and the basal ganglia within the brain. Serotonin and dopamine are the primary neurotransmitters for the neural circuits that connect these areas.

Serotonin is one of the major neurotransmitters within the brain.[153] Relatively high concentrations of serotonin are present in the *hypothalamus* and the basal ganglia. A variety of physiological functions are modulated by serotonin, including pain perception; aggressive, sexual, and impulsive behaviors; mood, anxiety; and sleep, temperature, appetite, movement, and balance.[153, 154]

hypothalamus — a small brain structure critically involved in survival functions, such as: temperature regulation, heart rate, blood pressure, feeding behavior, water intake, and emotional and sexual behavior

Although OCD has historically been linked to abnormal serotonin function, "The Serotonin Hypothesis of OCD" is based primarily on the finding that medications effective in treating OCD are limited to antidepressants with potent or selective effects on serotonin neurotransmission.[118, 155–159]

Research results suggest that serotonin function is abnormal in OCD and that successful treatment with serotonin reuptake inhibitor (SRI) medications appears to "correct" this abnormality.[155, 157–162] Interestingly, manipulating the amount of serotonin available during SRI treatment can induce a relapse. This suggests that the therapeutic benefits achieved by the SRI medications in OCD depend on serotonin. At the same time, research indicates that the other neurotransmitters (norepinephrine and dopamine) appear to be normal in subjects with OCD, further confirming the unique importance of serotonin.[155, 158, 159, 163]

No specific test of serotonin levels can be used to diagnose OCD. In fact, most people with OCD have normal blood levels of serotonin.[118, 155, 159, 164] Moreover, abnormal serotonin function can also be present in healthy volunteers without psychiatric symptoms as well as in subjects with depression, panic, anorexia, bulimia, or schizophrenia.[154] Since it is widely distributed and involved in so many different functions, the lack of consistent or specific serotonin abnormalities in OCD is not particularly surprising.[153] It is also possible that the abnormal findings involving serotonin in OCD do not really represent the main cause of OCD. Instead, perhaps serotonin is only secondarily involved in OCD. That is, the alterations in serotonin may well result from a genetic defect that increases vulnerability for OCD when serotonin abnormalities are present. So, while present in OCD, these abnormalities may not cause OCD.

Here's how the physiology of serotonin neurotransmission works:

neurons — nerve cells consisting of cell bodies or soma, axons

dendrites — small processes branching out from the neuron that detects electrical signals emitted by other neurons and transmits them to the cell body

synaptic cleft — gap between neurons

pre-synaptic neuron — area proximal to the synapse

post-synaptic neuron — area lying adjacent to the nerve terminal that contains the post-synaptic receptors

▶ *Neurons* (which relay signals from the soma to their terminals where they trigger the release of neurotransmitters) and *dendrites* (which receive messages from receptors and then transmit them to the soma) communicate by releasing neurotransmitters into the *synaptic cleft*.

▶ The *pre-synaptic neuron* is responsible for packaging, releasing, and delivering the neurotransmitter into the synapse, where it can diffuse across to the *post-synaptic neuron*.

▶ Neurotransmitters attach to a specific post-synaptic receptor, forming a temporary binding complex with the receptor, analogous to a "lock-and-key" formation.

▶ Binding of the messenger to the receptor results in a chemical change that leads to a biological response, such as a behavior, a thought, or a reaction.

▶ Once delivery of the message occurs, the receptor releases the neurotransmitter back into the synaptic cleft.

▶ Most neurotransmitters are subsequently re-absorbed by a specialized re-uptake site located on the pre-synaptic neuron, which is selective for serotonin, dopamine, or norepinephrine, respectively.

▶ Once the neurotransmitter re-enters the pre-synaptic side of the neuron, rapid destruction by enzymes such as monoamine oxidase (MAO) occurs. Enzymes are also present in the synapse to destroy neurotransmitters that are not immediately re-absorbed by the re-uptake pump mechanism.

Multiple points of regulation exist between the pre-synaptic and post-synaptic neurons. Incoming signals received by the post-synaptic receptor result in activation or inhibition of subsequent neuronal activity.

In this way, constant communication occurs between the pre- and post-synaptic neurons in an attempt to maintain homeostasis. For example, increasing amounts of serotonin within the synapse will trigger several reactions designed to "turn-off" or "reduce" further increases in serotonin.

What are the First-Line Medications Used to Treat OCD?

Medications effective for treating OCD are limited to antidepressants that potently or selectively block the serotonin re-uptake pump. Such medications are labeled serotonin re-uptake inhibiting (SRI) antidepressants and are considered the first-line medication treatments for OCD.[156, 165–168] SRIs are also considered effective for treating OCD in children.[169]

SRI antidepressants include the tricyclic antidepressant (TCA), clomipramine (Anafranil®), and the selective serotonin re-uptake inhibitor antidepressants (SSRIs). SSRI medications currently approved by the U.S. Federal Drug Administration (FDA) for the treatment of OCD include:

Despite SRI medications remaining the cornerstone of OCD treatment, renewed interest exists in other chemicals (e.g., neuropeptides and hormones). However, no consistent findings have yet emerged.

- ▶ Fluoxetine (Prozac®)
- ▶ Sertraline (Zoloft®)
- ▶ Paroxetine (Paxil®)
- ▶ Fluvoxamine (Luvox®)

Because SSRI medications do not directly influence other receptors or block the norepinephrine re-uptake pump mechanism, they have a relatively benign side effect and toxicity profile and are relatively safe in overdose. Except for fluoxetine, rapid discontinuation of SSRIs is also commonly associated with symptoms of withdrawal, which can persist for as long as one to two weeks.[170] Paroxetine is most frequently implicated in withdrawal symptoms.[171] However, similar symptoms can also occur with fluvoxamine and sertraline.

Note: *Allow at least four to six weeks before achieving a steady-state concentration with fluoxetine when initiating treatment or modifying the dose. When fluvoxamine doses exceed 150 mg/day, administer in two, divided doses/day.*

Typical SSRI withdrawal symptoms reported include dizziness, headache, tingling, "electric-shock" sensations, and flu-like symptoms.[170, 172] A single dose of the medication can be used to rapidly block withdrawal symptoms prior to re-instituting a more gradual tapering of the medication.

There are substantial differences in the side effect and safety profile of clomipramine versus the SSRI antidepressants. The table in figure 4.2 on page 62 highlights the main differences between the two and reports the drugs' mechanisms of action, common dosages, and side effects. The most serious side effects and special concerns are noted in bold print.[170]

Special concerns for clomipramine involve overdose potential and preexisting medical conditions. Doses should not exceed 250 mg/day because of link to an unacceptable seizure risk (1–3 percent). A five- to seven-day supply of clomipramine represents a potentially fatal overdose if taken at once. Caution should be taken for patients with pre-existing serious medical conditions, such as: heart disease, a seizure disorder, or certain types of

In spite of clomipramine's unparalleled track record of efficacy in OCD, its potential toxicity often results in it being relegated to a second line position in the initial treatment of OCD.

Figure 4.2 SRI Medication Treatment Overview

Name of Medication(s)	Mechanism of Action	Dose (mg/day)	Medication Half-Life

SRI Medication

Clomipramine (Anafranil®)[168, 169]	Clomipramine's benefit in OCD is linked to its effects on the serotonin re-uptake pump, but it also has several other chemical effects that may prove unwanted including, antihistamine and anticholinergic effects (see side effects).	150–250	Approximately a day (19–37 hrs.), so it can be effectively administered in a once-a-day dosing regimen (within the recommended dose range).

Common Side Effects

Side effects attributed to the anticholinergic and antihistamine properties of clomipramine include dry mouth, fatigue, sedation, tremor, dizziness, increased heart rate, constipation, and weight gain.[162, 165]

SSRI Medications

Fluoxetine (Prozac®)[168, 180–182]	Pharmacological effects are restricted to the selective blockade of the serotonin re-uptake pump.[165, 170, 198]	20–80	2–4 days for fluoxetine and 7–10 days for nor-fluoxetine (active metabolite)
Sertraline (Zoloft®)*[168, 183–187]		50–200	24 hours for sertraline and paroxetine
Paroxetine (Paxil®)[168, 188–194]		40–60	12–24 hours for fluvoxamine
Fluvoxamine (Luvox®)**[168, 195–197]		200–300	

Common Side Effects

All: Sexual dysfunction (decreased libido, delayed orgasm, or anorgasmia), decreased appetite, nausea, fatigue, daytime sedation, nervousness, restlessness, and anxiety

For fluoxetine: nervousness, agitation, anxiety, respiratory complaints, headache, nausea, dry mouth, and tremors

For sertraline: diarrhea, tremor, dry mouth, insomnia, decreased libido, nausea, anorexia, ejaculation failure, increased sweating, and increased weight gain

For paroxetine: sexual dysfunction, frequent urination, weakness, fatigue, dizziness, sweating, nausea, somnolence, headache, and constipation

For fluvoxamine: drowsiness, constipation, anorexia, insomnia, nausea, asthenia, somnolence, abnormal ejaculation, nervousness, and dry mouth

glaucoma. Seizures, abnormal heart rhythms, and coma can occur when ingesting a dose of clomipramine that is only four to six times the usual recommended daily dose.[152] Abrupt discontinuation of clomipramine is associated with withdrawal symptoms including headache, insomnia, increased salivation, flu-like symptoms, and diarrhea.

Citalopram (Celexa®) is a relatively new SSRI approved by the FDA for treating depression.[173] However, several studies suggest that citalopram is also effective for treating OCD, including pediatric OCD. There is also some initial data suggesting that citalopram may be effective in patients considered refractory to other standard OCD medication.[174–178] Additionally, results from a preliminary study of a mirtazapine-citalopram combination revealed an earlier reduction in OCD symptoms and fewer undesired side effects in comparison to citalopram therapy alone.[179] However, this study did not demonstrate any difference in overall longer-term response rate in the combined versus monotherapy groups.

Note that citalopram is not specifically FDA approved for treating OCD.

Half-Life and Dosing

The long *half-life* of fluoxetine has several important implications. Usually the time it takes for a medication to achieve a steady amount within the blood (steady-state concentration) is estimated by multiplying the half-life of the medication by five. Therefore, it takes four to six weeks before achieving a steady-state concentration with fluoxetine after initiating treatment or modifying the fluoxetine dose. Thus, changing the dose more often than every four to six weeks is unwise since the amount of fluoxetine available within the blood has not yet stabilized. Fluoxetine's long half-life also suggests that less-frequent doses may be possible in some patients without loss of effectiveness. Therefore, fluoxetine may be relatively advantageous for patients who often miss doses or are less likely to comply with daily dose regimens.[170, 198]

half-life — the time required to eliminate 50 percent of a medication from the body

Changes in dose for sertraline and paroxetine should reflect steady-state concentrations achieved within four to five days. Changes in dose for fluvoxamine should reflect the ability to stabilize within three to four days.

Important differences including optimal target dose and treatment response characteristics exist when SRI antidepressant medications are prescribed for the treatment of OCD versus depressive disorders.[166] In addition, the majority of medications that are FDA-approved in the treatment of depression are ineffective in the treatment of OCD. The lack of efficacy of most antidepressants in OCD has historically been attributed to their relative lack of potency and/or selectivity for the neurotransmitter serotonin; however it is important to note that this remains

See figure 4.2 for half-life indications of treatment medications.

unproven.[199] The five SRI medications listed in figure 4.2 on page 62 remain the only medications that are FDA-approved for OCD treatment in the U.S.[165]

The cardinal features of OCD pharmacotherapy include:

- ▶ Medication requires an extremely lengthy time period (often 6–10 weeks) before therapeutic effects occur.

- ▶ Symptom improvement in OCD is generally partial (25 to 40 percent), with remission being very rare (less than 10 percent).[48, 156, 165, 166, 200–202]

Due to the inherent delayed onset with SRIs in OCD, effective treatment should continue for at least a year.[156, 166] Patients with OCD generally remain improved as long as they continue taking SRI medications.[68, 186] There is some evidence that the SRI medication dose may be reduced after six to nine months in many patients without substantial loss of effectiveness. In fact, several studies have suggested that a 30 to 70 percent decrease in SRI dose is often possible after 9–12 months of treatment, without substantial loss of therapeutic effects.[203, 204]

The risk of withdrawal symptoms can be dramatically reduced if the dose is gradually reduced over several months. A reasonable rate of dose reduction is 50–100 mg. per month for clomipramine, fluvoxamine, or sertraline and 20 mg. per month for paroxetine. Due to its extensive half-life, however, fluoxetine can be discontinued without an extensive tapering regimen.[170]

Effectiveness of SRI Medications for Treating OCD

Overall, when comparing the various SRI treatments, researchers find similar effectiveness in reducing OCD symptoms (approximately a 30 percent reduction in symptoms from the pre-treatment baseline).[156, 158, 165–167, 201] Important differences exist (noted in the medication treatment chart on page 62) in specific dose recommendations among the SSRIs and in their use with children and adolescents.

It remains controversial whether clomipramine is more effective than the SSRIs for OCD, although most experts recommend a trial of clomipramine before considering a patient to be refractory to medication or "giving up" on medication treatment. That is, clomipramine should always be considered as a first-line OCD treatment option along with the SSRIs.

Systematic data concerning the potential rate of "cross-response" between individual SRI medications is limited. A preliminary uncontrolled trial conducted with 81 patients with OCD involved separate trials of clomipramine and fluoxetine, respectively. Results included: [112, 166]

- ▶ Approximately 65 percent of the patients who improved with clomipramine also responded to subsequent treatment with fluoxetine.

- ▶ Patients who failed to respond to clomipramine were also unlikely to improve during a subsequent trial of fluoxetine therapy.

▶ Eighty percent of patients who responded to fluoxetine also responded to subsequent clommipramine treatment.

Overall, research on the effectiveness of SRI treatment of OCD indicates that:

▶ Clomipramine and the SSRIs are similarly effective and considered first-line treatment for OCD.

▶ SSRI medications have an improved side effect and safety profile in comparison to clomipramine.

Many people with OCD will fail to respond to one SRI medication, but will experience substantial improvement when treated with a different SRI. Nonetheless, as many as 20–25 percent of those with OCD will not respond to any of the SRI medications.[57, 156, 166, 200–202] In addition, several factors (listed below) can result in a patient with OCD being erroneously labeled as "medication refractory" or "SRI resistant":[57, 156, 166, 200–202]

▶ Being treated initially with medications other than clomipramine or an SSRI (lack of SRI trials)

▶ Giving up too soon on a medication (taking an SRI less than a minimum of six to 10 weeks)

▶ Taking too low of a medication dose

▶ Being misdiagnosed

▶ Abusing alcohol or drugs

▶ Not taking medications as prescribed or routinely missing doses

▶ Having unreasonable expectations (e.g., expecting symptoms to rapidly improve or disappear)

Each of these factors should be considered, explored, and excluded when a patient with OCD fails to benefit from medication treatment. Before being considered as "resistant" to SRI medications, a patient should receive separate and adequate trials (lasting more than 10 weeks for each SRI) of at least three of the four SSRI medications (fluoxetine, fluvoxamine, sertraline, paroxetine) as well as a separate clomipramine trial.[57, 156, 166, 200–202]

In contrast to conventional wisdom as well as results associated with smaller trials, results from large, multicenter trials of sertraline and fluoxetine reported that only 20–30 percent of patients with OCD relapsed after discontinuation of their SSRI medication.[205, 206] Additional long-term, multicenter trials of sertraline, paroxetine, and fluoxetine conducted in patients with OCD have also reported similarly low relapse rates (10 to 20 percent) after SRI discontinuation.[207–209]

To minimize the risk of relapse, it is very important to slowly and gradually taper SRI medication rather than abruptly discontinue it. Concurrent use of behavior therapy may be particularly effective in preventing relapse after discontinuing medication.

Augmentation Strategies

Since medication response is usually partial, clinicians often turn to augmentation strategies as a means of optimizing the degree of OCD symptom improvement. The most common augmentation tactics reported in OCD involve combining an SRI with a second (augmenting) medication. Despite a plethora of case reports and open trials suggesting that a wide variety of medications will successfully augment SRI medications, results from controlled trials have been much less promising.

Several recent investigations, however, have revealed that the addition of an atypical antipsychotic medication may be a particularly promising strategy for patients with OCD who fail to adequately respond to an SRI medication.

SRI and Antipsychotic Medication Augmentation

Observations based on a number of research studies conducted over the past few years with antipsychotic medication, especially newer atypical antipsychotics, such as olanzapine (Zyprexa®), risperidone (Risperdal®), and quetiapine (Seroquel®), suggest that antipsychotic medication may be effective as adjunctive therapy (not as monotherapy) for treating OCD, especially for patients having an inadequate response to SRIs.[210–215] *Atypical antipsychotic* medications offer several treatment benefits: they are less likely to cause movement disorders than first-generation antipsychotics, improve social withdrawal and flat affect, and have a much better overall safety profile.

atypical antipsychotics — newer, or second-generation, antipsychotic medications typically used to treat schizophrenia and other psychoses

Augmentation strategies may also be particularly effective in patients with:

- ▶ **Co-existing or persistent depression —** Augmentation with lithium (Eskalith®) may be helpful in improving the depressive symptoms.[156, 166]

- ▶ **Co-existing Tourette's or tic disorders —** Adding in a low dose of neuroleptic medication [e.g., haloperidol (Haldol®) or pimozide (Orap®)] to an SRI may help to improve OCD and suppress tics.[216] Moreover, preliminary reports with risperidone added to an SRI medication suggest further improvement in OCD symptoms even in the absence of a co-existing tic disorder.[118, 217–219]

- ▶ **Persistent anxiety —** Adding in clonazepam (Klonopin®) or buspirone (BuSpar®) may help to reduce persistent or "breakthrough" anxiety symptoms, but is unlikely to produce further improvement in OCD symptoms.[220]

Particular subgroups of patients with OCD, such as those with comorbid tics and schizotypal personality disorder, may also be more likely to respond to augmentation with an antipsychotic medication.

What Other Medications are Used to Treat OCD?

Other agents used in OCD treatment include:

- **Cyclic antidepressants** — Despite encouraging case reports, trazodone (Desyrel®) was no more effective than a placebo in treating OCD.[221, 222] Mirtazapine (Remeron®), which is a tetracyclic antidepressant, has been found to enhance serotonergic function in a small, double-blind controlled study.[223]

- **Newer generation, non-SSRI antidepressants** — Venlafaxine (Effexor®) may be effective in OCD, although controlled studies have yielded mixed results.[192, 224–228] Venlafaxine has a similar, benign side effect and safety profile to the SSRI antidepressants.[226]

- **Anti-anxiety agents** — Controlled trials of buspirone (BuSpar®), clonazepam (Klonopin®), and oxazepam (Serax®) have largely failed to support their effectiveness, especially as monotherapy, in OCD. Clonazepam studies have produced mixed results.[220]

- **Combined SRI regimens** — Although combined clomipramine/SSRI or SSRI/SSRI regimens reportedly have widespread clinical use, controlled data is lacking. Given this as well as potential drug interactions, combining SSRIs or clomipramine plus an SSRI in OCD cannot be endorsed at this time.

- **MAOI antidepressants** — Patients with OCD who also have severe panic attacks, social phobia, or prominent obsessions about illness, especially bowel complaints (e.g., constipation), may represent a sub-group likely to respond to MAOI treatment.[166, 201, 229, 230] It is important to be very cautious, however, when considering MAOI treatment since numerous and potentially fatal food and drug interactions have been identified.[231] Additionally, MAOIs require an extensive "washout period" after SRI discontinuation. In general, MAOI antidepressants, phenelzine (Nardil®), or tranylcypromine (Parnate®), do not appear to be effective for most people with OCD.[156] While limited evidence exists that phenelzine may help some patients with prominent symmetry obsessions, increasingly few physicians in the U.S. feel comfortable or have experience prescribing MAOI antidepressants.[167]

> *MAOI use for patients with OCD should likely be restricted to those who fail to respond to SRIs and have access to a clinician experienced in dealing with MAOI treatment issues.*

What Other Biologically Based Treatments are Available for OCD?

Other treatments used to reduce OCD symptoms include neurosurgery and electroconvulsive therapy (ECT) as well as transcranial magnetic stimulation (TMS) and deep brain stimulation (DBS).

Neurosurgery

Neurosurgery should only be considered an option for patients with severe, incapacitating OCD symptoms failing to respond to multiple and adequate treatment trials that include SRI medication and behavioral therapy.[167] Clinicians typically do not consider neurosurgery unless a patient with OCD fails to respond to or tolerate:

- At least three separate and adequate SSRI trials
- An adequate trial of clomipramine
- An adequate trial of behavioral therapy (exposure and response prevention)
- Two or more augmentation strategies (e.g., clonazepam, risperidone)
- Non-SRI antidepressant trial (e.g., venlafaxine, mirtazapine)

In neurosurgery, surgeons create microscopic lesions in specific brain areas implicated as functionally abnormal in OCD. These lesions are localized to the sites that contain the neural pathways that connect the frontal cortex to the limbic and basal ganglia structures and are thought to partly correct an abnormally overactive circuit. Although several different surgical procedures exist, *cingulotomy* and *capsulotomy* are the two, most common ones used in OCD. Results from long-term, follow-up studies of patients with OCD reveal that:

cingulotomy — removal of the mid-line fold in the outer layer of both sides of the brain, which contain neural pathways from the cortex to the inner brain

capsulotomy — removal of the front part of the internal capsule of the brain, which contains nerves that connect the cerebral cortex to the basal ganglia

- At an average follow-up time of 32 months after one or more cingulotomies for treatment-refractory OCD, 32 percent (14/44) of patients were responders and 14 percent (6/44) were partial responders.[232]
- Two and one-half years after cingulotomy, 28 percent (5/18) of previously refractory patients were responders, and 17 percent (3/18) were partial responders.[233]
- In 26 patients followed for a mean of 10 years after a cingulotomy, 38 percent had substantial improvement, whereas the remainder were considered unchanged (46 percent) or worse (15 percent) after the procedure.[234]
- After capsulotomy, 48 percent (9/19) of patients with OCD twere rated as improved. Lesions created within

the right internal capsule appeared to be associated with the most favorable outcome.[235]

► Seizures (five percent) or infection (one percent) are rare after neurosurgery.[201, 233–235]

► No difference can be detected in personality or intellectual and memory functions after neurosurgery; however, subtle differences occur on the Wisconsin Card Sorting Test that assesses frontal lobe function.[151, 152, 233]

These results suggest that 25 to 30 percent of patients with OCD who previously were refractory to multiple treatment interventions may improve with neurosurgery. However, all reported studies have been uncontrolled and have included relatively few patients. With these issues in mind, further research is needed before neurosurgery can be considered anything but a last-resort option.

Electroconvulsive Therapy (ECT)

ECT is used to elicit a grand mal seizure by controlled electrical stimulation. Although ECT is a highly effective treatment for severe depression, it is rarely effective for OCD.[236]

Typically ineffective for most patients with OCD, isolated reports suggest that ECT may be beneficial for some.[237] As a result, ECT should only be considered for patients who have:[156, 201]

► Severe, co-existing depression complicated by psychotic features or suicidal ideation

► Failed to respond to standard treatment interventions, including medication and behavioral therapy

Transcranial Magnetic Stimulation (TMS)

TMS is a technique currently being studied primarily for the treatment of affective disorders. This technology uses a magnetic field to alter neurotransmission in focal areas of the cortex and can be applied to target frontal regions implicated in OCD pathophysiology. Preliminary data suggests that TMS administered to lateral prefrontal regions may prove effective in some patients with OCD who fail to respond to standard OCD treatments.[167]

Deep Brain Stimulation (DBS)

DBS involves implanting and "turning on" electrodes in specific areas of the brain to chronically stimulate or inhibit surrounding tissue. Used for Parkinson's disease, DBS treatment has had positive (but very preliminary) success with treatment-resistant OCD.[167] Especially promising is the fact that DBS causes less intra-cerebral neuronal damage than neurosurgery.[168]

How Effective are Medications vs. Behavior Therapy for Treating OCD?

In the ongoing debate about the efficacy of medications versus psychotherapy, these factors are critical:

▶ Early (acute) treatment results, short-term gains, and relapse rates

▶ Treatment compliance (willingness to take medications with sometimes intolerable side effects versus ability to comply with the demands of exposure treatment)

▶ Cost considerations

▶ Type of symptoms

Early (Acute) Treatment Results, Short-term Gains, and Relapse Rates

OCD treatment outcome research has primarily compared results of behavior therapy (especially exposure and response prevention) with SRI medication. Both yield gains in short-term treatment of six months or less. Exposure and response prevention studies have found that 90 percent of patients experienced at least moderate improvement after treatment. At the time of follow-up evaluation (months to several years), 76 percent remained improved.[57] SRI medication is similarly effective with 65 to 80 percent of patients improving immediately after treatment.[48, 202]

Recent studies also support the use of cognitive behavior/behavior therapy as more effective than medications alone.[238–240] One study found that solution-focused brief therapy (SFBT) combined with paroxetine was more effective than paroxetine alone.[241]

However, follow-up studies with drug therapy are not as promising. Several studies indicate as many as 90 percent of medication responders relapse within four weeks of discontinuing SRI medication.[203] Therefore, researchers consider behavior therapy as the first-line option for treating OCD and find it particularly essential as an add-on treatment for patients taking medications, especially those considering discontinuation of medication.[156 167, 242–244]

Education and information about OCD and effective treatments represents one of the most important components in maximizing a successful treatment.

Treatment Compliance

Sometimes-intolerable side effects often make medication less desirable than exposure and response prevention. SRI antidepressants are valuable for patients who either refuse or fail to respond to exposure treatment. Conversely, exposure therapy may help patients taking medications maintain their treatment gains or may be preferable to experiencing some side effects.

Therefore, combining SRI antidepressants and exposure and response prevention seems to facilitate one another with many patients and may be the best available treatment for most people with OCD.[57]

Clomipramine, along with exposure therapy, may offer an additional benefit over clomipramine alone in reducing OCD symptoms.[246]

Cost Considerations

Initially, medications are more cost-effective than psychotherapy. However, the higher relapse rates associated with OCD medication treatment may necessitate long-term and perhaps even life-long medication treatment or added behavior therapy to prevent relapse. Though OCD medication treatment is less expensive in the short-term, behavioral therapy may be more cost-effective over time.

Symptom Types

Symptom-related factors may partially suggest why the results achieved with behavior therapy exceed those attained with medication treatment in OCD. For example, subjects with primary cleaning or checking ritual symptoms are over-represented in OCD behavioral therapy studies, and extraordinary success rates are often achieved when such patients receive behavior therapy. However, controversy exists as to whether or not the results from behavioral therapy studies are applicable to the majority of those suffering from OCD. In particular, there is very limited data concerning the success rate for behavior therapy in those with OCD who have only obsessions or who exhibit less common compulsions (e.g., hoarding, counting, or symmetry/completeness).[57, 200, 201, 245]

In contrast, patients with a wide array of OCD symptoms, including the more difficult-to-treat symptoms of hoarding, counting, and perfectionism, are routinely included in medication studies. This may explain in part the reduced, long-term success rate associated with medication treatment.

With these issues in mind, combined medication and behavior therapy, which is currently receiving significant research attention, probably represents the most effective OCD treatment, especially in children.[241, 247, 248] Research results confirm that the same biochemical changes occur after either medication or behavioral therapy.[43, 44] Additionally, combining cognitive-behavioral therapy, which includes exposure and response prevention, and SRI medication appears to reduce OCD symptoms more than no treatment or either treatment administered alone.[249]

Key Concepts for Chapter Four:

1. OCD may be related to a spectrum of other disorders (e.g., Tourette's syndrome) that share some of the same vulnerability genes.

2. About 40 percent of those suffering from OCD have a biological relative with OCD. Additionally, identical twins are more likely to have OCD symptoms than fraternal twins.

3. Neuroimaging studies indicate that successful treatment — with either behavior therapy or medication, or both — normalizes brain activity.

4. OCD has been linked to abnormal serotonin function; antidepressants with potent or selective effects on serotonin neurotransmission appear to correct these abnormalities.

5. SRIs (clomipramine, fluoxetine, sertraline, paroxetine, and fluvoxamine) are first-line medications for OCD. Of those, clomipramine is recommended less since the others have more favorable side effect and safety profiles.

6. SRI therapy should not be abandoned until at least three separate SSRIs and a clomipramine trial have been completed, unless the patient cannot tolerate SRI side effects.

7. The most promising medication augmentation strategies use atypical antipsychotic medications with SRI treatment.

Appendix:
Assessment Measures

BSESSIVE compulsive disorder (OCD) assessment measures include:

- ▶ Patient-rated self-report instruments
- ▶ Structured interviews
- ▶ Psychometric assessments

Patient-Rated Self-Report Instruments

Patient-rated, self-report instruments particularly useful for diagnosing OCD include:

- ▶ Obsessive Compulsive Inventory-Short Version (OCI-SV)
- ▶ Padua Inventory (PI)
- ▶ Yale-Brown Obsessive Compulsive Checklist and Scale — Self-Report form (Y-BOCS) (see information on pages 75–76)
- ▶ Vancouver Obsessional Compulsive Inventory (VOCI)

OCI-SV

The OCI is an 18-item measure that addresses six subscales:

1. Washing
2. Checking/doubting
3. Ordering
4. Obsessing
5. Hoarding
6. Mental neutralizing

The instrument has shown excellent internal consistency (.82 – .90) in patients with OCD as well as good test-retest reliability. OCI-SV subscales appear to have particularly good sensitivity and specificity for distinguishing those with OCD from nonclinical participants. It is particularly useful because of its subscale containing items that assess all three compulsive hoarding components.[250]

Padua Inventory (PI)

Published by Italian researchers in 1988, the PI consists of 60 items that assess common obsessive and compulsive symptoms and the degree to which they interfere with daily functioning.[251] Each item is rated on a five-point scale and measures the degree of disturbance brought on by a thought or behavior. The scores range from 0 (not at all) to 4 (very much). The total score range is from 0 to 240.

Other patient-rated, self-report assessments are not as comprehensive in assessing OCD symptoms; these include:

- ▶ *Symptom Checklist-90 (SCL-90) — Only one very brief subscale among many that measures obsessive or compulsive symptoms*

- ▶ *Leyton Obsessional Inventory (LOI) — Provides a narrow focus on OCD, mostly on contamination/cleaning symptoms*

73

It is important to consider cultural factors that may influence responses to test items. For example, one large analysis found differences in scores on every factor of the PI between White and Black participants. Study authors found these differences reflected extraneous factors, perhaps related to cultural practices and the fear of being negatively stereotyped.[252]

The PI measures symptoms using four scales:

1. **Contamination** — The Contamination Scale contains typical washing and cleaning compulsions. It includes statements, such as "I avoid public telephones because I am afraid of contagion or disease."

2. **Checking** — The Checking Scale measures typical checking and repeating compulsions. A representative statement is: "I check and recheck gas and water taps and light switches after turning them off."

3. **Mental control** — The Mental Control scale measures ability to control, suppress, or ignore obsessive thoughts and includes an assessment of certainty or doubt. Statements include, "I invent doubts and problems about most of the things I do," "I worry about remembering completely unimportant things and make an effort not to forget them," or "When I start thinking of certain things, I become obsessed with them."

4. **Impulses** — The Impulses scale assesses concern about harming others due to carelessness, lack of preparation, loss of self-control, or inability to provide a safe environment.

validity — the extent to which the test actually measures what it claims to measure

The PI has demonstrated satisfactory reliability and *validity*.[38] As a result, it is increasingly utilized in research studies.[38]

Currently, the PI and OCI-SV are more commonly used than other self-report instruments.

VOCI

An updated version of the Maudsley Obsessional Compulsive Inventory (MOCI), the VOCI is a 55-item measurement for a wide array of obsessions, compulsions, avoidance behavior, and personality characteristics common with OCD. The items in the VOCI are grouped into subscales for Contamination, Checking, Obsession, Hoarding, Just Right, and Indecisiveness. Scoring is done on a five-point Likert scale, with total scores and subscales computed by summing all items (possible total scores range from 0 to 212).

Shown to be reliable and valid, the VOCI may be more useful in the primary care setting than other OCD instruments due to a shorter administrative time (five minutes).[253]

Structured Interviews

Structured interviews include:

- ▶ Structured Clinical Interview for the DSM-IV (SCID)
- ▶ Anxiety Disorders Interview Schedule-Revised (ADIS-R)
- ▶ Yale-Brown Obsessive Compulsive Scale and Symptom Checklist — Interview version (Y-BOCS)

Structured Clinical Interview for the DSM-IV (SCID) and Anxiety Disorders Interview Schedule-Revised (ADIS-R)

Many clinicians use structured interview techniques to diagnose OCD in clinical or community samples, especially the SCID and the ADIS-R.[254, 255] These interviews are often time-consuming and difficult to use in clinical practice and tend to be used mainly for research purposes.

Trained interviewers use the SCID and the ADIS to ensure a structured and consistent format for identifying the presence of psychiatric symptoms. Both instruments require an hour or less to administer the OCD section, and they reliably diagnose OCD according to DSM-IV (TR) criteria. However, in each case, more time is required to complete the entire interview for all psychiatric disorders.[38]

No data exists comparing these two interviews. Clinicians generally prefer the ADIS because it more thoroughly details and quantifies OCD symptoms, especially insight into obsessive fears, resistance, and avoidance. Both instruments may be used *formally* to diagnose OCD or *informally* during initial clinical interviews to identify major OCD symptoms.

formally — strictly following the order of questions

informally — the evaluator asks only those questions believed to pertain to that individual patient

Yale-Brown Obsessive Compulsive Scale (Y-BOCS)

Perhaps the most useful structured interview tool for clinicians to use in rating a patient's obsessive and compulsive behavior is the Yale-Brown Obsessive Compulsive Scale (Y-BOCS), published in 1989.[256] To use the Y-BOCS, the clinician initially reads definitions and examples of obsessions and compulsions to the patient. Then, the clinician asks about past or current experience with 36 specific obsessions and 23 specific rituals on a checklist, containing the following general categories.[38]

- ▶ Aggressive/harming
- ▶ Contamination
- ▶ Sexual
- ▶ Hoarding/saving
- ▶ Religious
- ▶ Symmetry/exactness
- ▶ Somatic
- ▶ Miscellaneous

The Y-BOCS has become the "gold standard" for assessing OCD in treatment outcome studies.[38]

Assessment of the patient's answers is far more comprehensive with the Y-BOCS than with other OCD instruments. Ten questions (five concerning obsessions; five about compulsions) assess OCD symptom severity in terms of five aspects of OCD pathology: time spent, interference, distress, resistance, and perceived control

Each of the 10 questions are scored on a scale from 0 (no symptoms) to 4 (extreme symptoms). The totals are added to yield a total score ranging from 0 to 40. Scores of 8–15 are considered mild, 16–23 moderate, 24–31 severe, and 32–40 extreme.

For adults, two modified versions of the Y-BOCS have been developed that reduce the time and ultimately the costs associated with this comprehensive assessment. These two versions are:

▶ **The self-report version** of the Y-BOCS is very similar to the original Y-BOCS, but allows patients to fill out the questionnaire on their own. This approach reduces costs because administration does not require the presence of the clinician.

▶ **The computer-assisted, telephone-administered version** of the Y-BOCS utilizes digitized human speech over the phone to provide a reliable, low-cost method capable of generating immediate scores. Unfortunately, this approach requires patients to be comfortable using a computer and to use the clinic's computer to complete the interview.

For children and adolescents, the Children's Yale-Brown Obsessive Compulsive scale (also available in a Spanish version) has proven to be a reliable and valid instrument for assessing childhood obsessions and compulsions.[252, 257] Recent research with children and adolescents aged 4–18 diagnosed with OCD indicates that the CY-BOCS showed good internal consistency and test-retest reliability on both obsession and compulsion severity scores as well as total scores for the instrument.[257] Additionally, the CY-BOCS results strongly correlated with clinician-rated measures of impairment, obsessions, and compulsions.[257]

The original Y-BOCS demonstrated very good *criterion-related validity* as well as *convergent validity*. The computer-administered and self-report versions also perform well in these areas, but require further evaluation.[41, 257, 258] The Y-BOCS is most useful for quantifying the level or severity of obsessive compulsive symptoms and measuring response to treatment.[41] Its two main weaknesses are being designed to assess OCD symptom severity, not to diagnose the disorder and being time consuming, requiring approximately 45 minutes to one hour to administer.

Glossary

A

amygdala — one of the basal ganglia that is part of the limbic system and believed to be involved in impulsivity and other functions

anoxia — brain cell death resulting from interruption of oxygen supply to the brain

antibodies — complex protein molecules created specifically to destroy organisms deemed to be dangerous

antibody titer — the dilution of a serum containing a specific antibody at which the solution just retains a specific activity (as neutralizing or precipitating an antigen), which it loses at any greater dilution

atypical antipsychotics — newer, or second-generation, antipsychotic medications typically used to treat schizophrenia and other psychoses

aversion relief — the process of punishing behavior followed by the ending of the punishment when the person stopped thinking the undesired thoughts or displaying undesired behaviors

B

basal ganglia — brain area comprised of several structures (including the caudate nucleus, putamen, and substantia nigra) that has a primary function to initiate and control body movements

body dysmorphic disorder — a mental disorder that involves a disturbed body image

C

capsulotomy — removal of the front part of the internal capsule of the brain, which contains nerves that connect the cerebral cortex to the basal ganglia

CAT (Computer Axial Tomography) scans — computer-assisted x-rays

caudate nucleus — a basal ganglia component involved in the voluntary control of movement

cingulotomy — removal of the mid-line fold in the outer layer of both sides of the brain, which contain neural pathways from the cortex to the inner brain

compulsions — acts the person performs over and over again, often according to certain "rules"

controlled research studies — research studies in which the various treatments in the study are regulated so that causal factors can be unambiguously identified

convergent validity — the relationship of a test to independent measures of the same trait

corrective emotional experience — when a patient reexperiences with the clinician an old, chronic conflicting pattern of behavior, such as extreme dependency, and the therapeutic relationship allows for a different healing outcome to the old pattern of behavior

criterion-related validity — the extent to which a measure of an attribute demonstrates an association with some independent or external indicator of that same attribute

77

D

dendrites — small processes branching out from the neuron that detects electrical signals emitted by other neurons and transmits them to the cell body

dizygotic — fraternal or non-identical twin derived from separate eggs and possessing different genetic characteristics

E

ego strength — self-confidence, resourcefulness, stability, and ability to cope with problems and stresses in life situations

encephalitis — viral infection of the brain leading to inflammation

etiology — the cause of a disorder

exposure and response prevention — the patient confronts obsessional cues and is prevented from performing compulsions

F

formally — strictly following the order of questions

G

gene — DNA sequence located at a specific site on a chromosome that codes for a certain characteristic(s); the biological basis of heredity

genetic link — tendency for genes to be inherited together despite coding for separate characteristics and being located on different chromosome locations.

group cohesiveness — the degree to which group members work together for the benefit of each other and the group as a whole

H

habituation — gradual, naturally occurring reduction of anxiety or discomfort over time, if exposure is maintained

half-life — the time required to eliminate 50 percent of a medication from the body

hallucinations — false sensory perceptions

hypnotics — medications that promote sleep

hypothalamus — a small brain structure critically involved in survival functions, such as: temperature regulation, heart rate, blood pressure, feeding behavior, water intake, and emotional and sexual behavior

I

imagined exposure — exposure to the feared stimuli through the use of mental imagery

imagined flooding — a clinical procedure where the clinician helps the patient repeatedly visualize being exposed to a certain obsessive cue without ritualizing until that cue or situation no longer evokes anxiety or discomfort

inappropriate affect — mood incongruent with context of a situation

informally — the evaluator asks only those questions believed to pertain to that individual client

insight — self-awareness or self-understanding of the underlying dynamics of one's actions

interpreting — the clinician reflects to the patient hypotheses regarding the connection between unconscious material and current or conscious feelings or behavior

in-vivo exposure — exposure to the actual anxiety-eliciting stimulus, such as a garbage can

irrational beliefs — false perceptions of reality based on exaggerated ex pectations

L

limbic system — brain region involved in smell, automatic behaviors, and emotions that surrounds the midbrain and has extensive connections with the thalamus and brain stem

loosening of associations — an individual's speech slips off the track from one topic to another

M

meta-analysis — a study of the collective findings of many individual outcome studies to give an overall level of effectiveness for a certain type of treatment

modeling — a technique where the clinician demonstrates exposure for the patient

monozygotic — derived from the same fertilized egg and identical genetic make-up

N

negative automatic thoughts — immediate interpretations about the meaning of obsessive thoughts

neurons — nerve cells consisting of cell bodies or soma, axons

neurotransmitters — chemical messengers that transmit signals from one nerve cell to another to ellicit physiological responses

O

obsessions — thoughts, images, or impulses that occur over and over again and feel out of one's control

over-valued ideation — belief that obsessive fears are realistic

P

PANDAS — complication of untreated strept throat where the streptococcus bacteria invades the brain in children/adolescents and results in damage to the basal ganglia region, producing OCD symptoms

paradoxical intention — a technique where the clinician instructs the patient to do more of the obsessions or compulsions

PET — Positron Emission Tomography

pheochromocytoma — a ususally benign tumor that causes increased secretion of epinephrine or norepinephrine

porphyria — a disorder involving the metabolism of phrphyrin — the foundation structure of hemoglobin, chlorophyll, and certain enzymes

positive transference — the patient recalls and relives pleasant experiences, feelings, and memories from the past as if they were occurring in the present

Post-encephalitic Parkinsonism — rigidity, tremor, and abnormally slow movements that develop as a result of encephalitis lethargica or "sleeping sickness"

post-synaptic neuron — area lying adjacent to the nerve terminal that contains the post-synaptic receptors

pre-synaptic neuron — area proximal to the synapse

prognosis — outcome in the future

progressive supranuclear palsy — genetic/familial condition characterized by deterioration of the brain cells in the cerebral cortex, basal ganglia, and other upper motor areas and resulting in weakness and/or paralysis

psychometric instruments — tests that measure psychological factors, such as personality, intelligence, beliefs, and fears

R

receptors — membrane-bound protein molecules with highly specific shapes that function as "landing" sites for specific chemical messengers (neurotransmitters or medications)

response prevention — deliberate blocking of overt and mental rituals and obsessive avoidance behaviors

S

satiation — a clinical procedure where the clinician has the patient verbalize ruminations while the clinician encourages the patient through the use of verbal prompts

schizotypal personality disorder — a personality disorder characterized by markedly eccentric and erratic thought, speech, and behavior as well as a tendency to withdraw from other people

sedatives — medications that help suppress anxiety by calming agitation and relaxing muscles

serotonergic medication — medications that specifically affect the neurotransmitter serotonin

serotonin hypothesis — the theory that impaired serotonin neurotransmission in the brain relates to OCD development

social phobia — a disorder characterized by episodes of panic anxiety in social settings, due to excessive concern about public embarrassment or possible adverse scrutiny

Socratic questioning — posing a series of questions to force the patient to defend irrational beliefs, such as: "What evidence do you have to support that idea? What's the likelihood of such an outcome? What are other possible explanations?"

SPECT — Single Photon Emission Computerized Tomography

state like — circumstance-dependent characteristic

Subjective Units of Distress (SUDs) scale — a scale ranging from 10–100 with 10 being the least anxiety provoking and 100 being the most anxiety provoking, which allows patients to express exactly how upsetting or distressing certain stimuli are in comparison to other anxiety experiences

Sydenham's chorea — rheumatic fever that spreads into the brain and damages the basal ganglion, resulting in involuntary, irregular (choreoathetoid) muscle movements of the face, neck, and limbs

synaptic cleft — gap between neurons

systematic desensitization — a clinical technique that pairs relaxation with imagery of anxiety-eliciting situations

T

thalamus — brain area with multiple connections to other brain regions that primarily functions as a relay station for body sensations, including pain and temperature

thought stopping — disrupting thoughts by having the person use the word or image, "Stop!" immediately following the thought to be prevented

thought insertion — the belief that some other being is placing thoughts in one's mind

Tourette's syndrome — neurological disorder characterized by semi-voluntary motor tics and vocalizations

trait like — permanent, inherent characteristic

trichotillomania — a disorder characterized by a repeated urge to pull out scalp, facila, or body hair as well as eyelashes

V

validity — the extent to which the test actually measures what it claims to measure

References

1. American Psychiatric Association (2000). *Diagnostic and statistical manual of mental disorders (4th ed. Text Revision)*. Washington, DC: American Psychiatric Association.

2. U.S. Census Bureau, Population Division (2005). http://www.census.gov/population/www/popclockus.html.

3. Harvard Health Publications, Harvard Medical School (2005). Obsessive-compulsive disorder: Battling persistent unwanted thoughts and senselessly repeated actions. *Harvard Mental Health Letter, 22(4)*.

4. Barlow, D.H., Durand, V.M. (2005). *Abnormal psychology: An integrative approach*. United States: Thomson/Wadsworth.

5. Riggs, D.S., and Foa, E.B. (1993). Obsessive compulsive disorder. In D.H. Barlow (Ed.). *Clinical handbook of psychological disorders*. New York: Guilford.

6. Flament, M.F. and Cohen, D. (2000). Child and adolescent obsessive-conpulsive disorder: A review. In Mario Maj, Norman Sartorius, et al (Eds.). Obsessive-compulsive disorder. *WPA series evidence and experience in psychiatry, 4*. New York: John Wiley and Sons.

7. National Institute of Mental Health. (2000). *Facts about obsessive-compulsive disorder* (Publication No. OM-99-4154). Bethesda, MD: NIMH Anxiety Disorders Education Program.

8. Piacentini, J., Langley, A.K., (2004). Cognitive-behavioral therapy for chikdren who have obsessive-compulsive disorder. *Journal of Clinical Psychology, 60(11)*: 1181–1194.

9. Abramowitz, J.S., Whiteside, S.P., Deacon, B.J. (2005). The effectiveness of treatment for pediatric obsessive-compulsive disorder: A meta-analysis. *Behavior Therapy, 36(1)*: 55–63.

10. Franklin, M., Foa, E., March, J.S. (2003). The pediatric obsessive-compulsive disorder treatment study: Rationale, design, and methods. *Journal of Child & Adolescent Psychopharmacology, 13(2, Suppl)*: S39–S51.

11. De Haan, E., Huyser, C., Boer, F. (2005). Obsessive-compulsive disorder in children and adolescents. *Tijdschrift voor Psychiatrie, 47(4)*: 229–238.

12. Heyman, I., Fombonne, E., Simmons, H., Ford, T., Meltzer, H., and Goodman, R. (2001). Prevalence of obsessive-compulsive disorder in the british nationwide survey of child mental health. *British Journal of Psychiatry*, 179(4), 324-329.

13. Rachman, S.J. (1985). An overview of clinical and research issues in obsessional-compulsive disorders. In M. Mavissakalia, S.M. Turner, and L. Michelson (Eds.). *Obsessive-compulsive disorder: Psychological and pharmacological treatment*. New York: Plenum Press.

14. Morrison, J. (1995). *DSM-IV made easy: The clinician's guide to diagnosis*. New York: Guilford Press.

15. Neal-Barnett, A.M. (2002). *OC multi-cultural issues*. http://www.ocfoundation.org/ocf_0010.htm

16. Koran, L.M., Thienemann, M.L., and Davenport, R. (1966). Quality of life for patients with obsessive-compulsive disorder. *American Journal of Psychiatry, 153*, 783-788.

17. Steketee, G. (1997). Disability and family burden in obsessive compulsive disorder. *Canadian Journal of Psychiatry, 42*, 919-928.

18. Greist, J.H. and Jefferson, J.W. (1995). Obsessive compulsive disorder. In G.O. Gabbard (Ed.) *Treatment of Psychiatric Disorders (2nd ed.)* (pp. 1477-1498).

19. Stanley, M.A. and Turner, S.M. (1995). Current status of pharmacological and behavioral treatment of obsessive-compulsive disorder. *Behavior Therapy, 26*, 163-186.

20. Taylor, S. (2002). Cognitions in obsessive compulsive disorder: An overview. In R.O. Frost and G. Steketee (Eds.), *Cognitive approaches to obsessive compulsive disorder: Theory, assessment and treatment*. Oxford: Elsevier.

21. Foa, E.B. and Kozak, M.J. (1986). Emotional processing of fear: Exposure to corrective information. *Psychological Bulletin, 99*, 20-35.

22. Lyoo, K., Lee, D.W., Kim, Y.S., Kong, S.W., Kwon, J.S. (2001). Patterns of temperament and character in subjects with obsessive-compulsive disorder. *Journal of Clinical Psychiatry, 62*, 637-641

23. Cottraux, J. and Gerard, D. (1998). Neuroimaging and neuroanatomical issues in OCD. In R. Swinson, M. Antony, S. Rachman and M. Richter (Eds.) *OCD: Theory, research, and treatment* (pp. 154-180). New York: The Guilford Press.

24. Cummings, J.L. and Cunningham, K. (1992). Obsessive-compulsive disorder in Huntington's disease. *Biological Psychiatry, 31(3)*, 263-70.

25. Rauch, S.L. and Jenike, M.A. (1993). Neurobiological models of obsessive-compulsive disorder. *Psychosomatics, 34(1)*, 20-32.

26. Allen, A., Leonard, H., and Swedo, S. (1995). Case study: A new infection-triggered, autoimmune subtype of pediatric OCD and Tourette's syndrome. *Journal of the American Academy of Child and Adolescent Psychiatry, 34(3)*, 307-311.

27. Kettle, P. and Marks, I. (1986). Neurological factors in obsessive-compusive disorder: Two case reports and a review of the literature. *British Journal of Psychiatry, 149*, 315-319.

28. Miguel-Filho, E. (1995). Obsessive-compulsive disorder and the basal ganglia. *Arq-Neuropsiquiatr, 53(4)*, 858-9.

29. Modell, J., Mountz, J., Curtis, G., and Greden, J. (1989). Neurophysiologic dysfunction in basal ganglia/limbic striatal and thalamocortical circuits as a pathogenetic mechanism of obsessive-compulsive disorder. *Journal of Neuro-psychiatry, 1*, 27-36.

30. Leonard, H.L. and Swedo, S.E. (2001). Paediatric autoimmune neuropsychiatric disorders associated with streptococcal infection (PANDAS). *International Journal of Neuropsychopharmacology, 4(2)*, 191-198.

31. Murphy, M.L. and Pichichero, M.E. (2002). Prospective identification and treatment of children with pediatric autoimmune neuropsychiatric disorder associated with group A streptococcal infection (PANDAS). *Archives of Pediatrics and Adolescent Medicine, 156(4)*, 356-361.

32. Steketee, G.S. (1993). *Treatment of obsessive-compulsive disorder.* New York: Guilford.

33. Steketee, G. and Pruyn, N.A. (1998). Families of individuals with OCD. In R. P. Swinson, M. M. Antony, S. J. Rachman, and M. A. Richters (Eds.) *Obsessive compulsive disorder: Theory, research, and treatment.* New York: Guilford.

34. Chambless, D. and Steketee, G. (1999). Expressed emotion and behavior therapy outcome: A prospective study with obsessive-compulsive and agoraphobic outpatients. *Journal of Consulting and Clinical Psychology, 67(5)*, 658-665.

35. Steketee, G., Van Noppen, B. (2003). Family approaches to treatment for obsessive compulsive disorder. *Journal of Family Psychotherapy, 14(4)*: 55–71.

36. Steketee, G., Van Noppen, B. (2003). Family responses and multifamily behavioral treatment for obsessive-compulsive disorder. *Brief Treatment & Crisis Intervention, 3(2)*: 231–247.

37. Tot, S., Yazici, K., Yazici, A., Erdem, P., et al. (2003). Factors associated with treatment response in obsessive compulsive disorder. *Anatolian Journal of Psychiatry, 4(4)*: 197–200.

38. Steketee, G. (1994). Behavioral assessment and treatment planning with obsessive compulsive disorder: A review emphasizing clinical application. *Behavior Therapy, 25*, 613-633.

39. Matsunaga, H., Kiriike, N., Matsui, T., Oya, K., Iwasaki, Y., Koshimune, K., Miyata, A., and Stein, D.J. (2002). Obsessive-compulsive disorder with poor insight. *Comprehensive Psychiatry, 43(2)*, 150-7.

40. Denys, D., de Geus, F., van Megen, H.J.G.M., Westenberg, H.G.M. (2004). Symptom dimensions in obsessive-compulsive disorder: Factor analysis on a clinician-rated scale and a self-report measure. *Psychopathology, 37(4)*: 181–189.

41. Taylor, S. (1995). Assessment of obsessions and compulsions: Reliability, validity, and sensitivity to treatment effects. *Clinical Psychology Review, 15*, 261-296.

42. Barrett, P., Healy, L., March, J.S. (2003). Behavioral avoidance test for childhood obsessive-compulsive disorder: A home-based observation. *American Journal of Psychotherapy, 1(80)*: 80–91.

43. Baxter, L.R., Schwartz, J.M., Bergman, K.S., Szubba, M.P., Guze, B.H., Mazziotta, J.C., Alazraki, A., Selin, C.E., Ferng, H.K., Munford, P., and Phelps, M.E. (1992). Caudate glucose metabolic rate changes with both drug and behavior therapy for obsessive-compulsive disorder. *Archives of General Psychiatry, 49*, 681-689.

44. Schwartz, J., Stoessel, P., Baxter, L., Martin, K., and Phelps, M. (1996). Systematic changes in cerebral glucose metabolic rate after successful behavior modification treatment of OCD. *Archives of General Psychiatry, 53*, 109-113.

45. Nakao, T., Nakagawa, A., Yoshiura, T., Nakatani, E., et al. (2005). Brain activation of patients with obsessive-compulsive disorder during neuropsychological and symptom provocation tasks before and after symptom improvement: A functional magnetic resonance imaging study. *Biological Psychiatry, 57(8)*: 901–910.

46. Foa, E.B., Steketee, G., and Ozarow, B.J. (1985). Behavior therapy with obsessive-compulsives: From theory to treatment. In M. Mavissakalian, S.M. Turner, and L. Michelson (Eds.) *Obsessive-compulsive disorder: Psychological and pharmacological treatments.* (pp. 49-120). New York: Plenum Press.

47. Meyer, V., Levy, R., and Schnurer, A. (1974). The behavioural treatment of obsessive-compulsive disorders. In H.R. Beech (Ed.) *Obsessional states.* (pp. 233-258). London: Methuen and Co.

48. Perse, T. (1988). Obsessive-compulsive disorder: A treatment review. *Journal of Clinical Psychiatry, 49*, 48-55.

49. Emmelkamp, P.M., and Kraanen, J. (1977). Therapist-controlled exposure in vivo versus self-controlled exposure in vivo: A comparison with obsessive-compulsive patients. *Behaviour Research and Therapy, 15(6)*, 491-495.

50. Taylor, S., Thordarson, D.S., Spring, T., Yeh, A.H., et al. (2003). Telephone-administered cognitive behavior therapy for obsessive-compulsive disorder. *Cognitive Behavior Therapy, 32(1)*: 13–25.

51. Clark, A., Kirkby, K.C., Daniels, BA., and Marks, I.M. (1998). A pilot study of computer-aided vicarious exposure for obsessive-compulsive disorder: Erratum. *Australian and New Zealand Journal of Psychiatry, 32(5)*, 740.

52. Osgood-Hynes, D.J., Greist, J.H., Marks, I.M., Baer, L., Heneman, S.W., Wenzel, K.W., Manzo, P.A., Parkin, J.R., Spierings, C.J., Dottl, S.L., and Vitse, H.M. (1998). Self-administered psychotherapy for depression using a telephone-accessed computer system plus booklets: An open U.S.-U.K. study. *Journal of Clinical Psychiatry, 59(7)*, 358-365.

53. Bachofen, M., Nakagawa, A., Marks, I.M., Park, J.M., Greist, J.H., Baer, L., Wenzel, K.W., Parkin, J.R., and Dottl, S.L. (1999). Home self-assessment and self-treatment of obsessive-compulsive disorder using a manual and a computer-conducted telephone interview: Replication of a UK-US study. *Journal of Clinical Psychiatry, 60(8)*, 545-549.

54. Nakagawa, A., Marks, I.M., Park, J.M., Bachofen, M., Baer, L., Dottl, S.L. and Greist, J.H. (2000). Self treatment of obsessive-compulsive disorder guided by manual and computer-conducted telephone interview. *Journal of Telemedicine and Telecare, 6(1)*, 22-26

55. Greist, J.H., Marks, I.M., Baer, L., Kobak, K.A., Wenzel, K.W., Hirsch, M.J., Mantle, J.M. and Clary, C.M. (2002). Behavior therapy for obsessive-compulsive disorder guided by a computer or by a clinician compared with relaxation as a control. *Journal of Clinical Psychiatry, 63(2)*, 138-145.

56. Greist, J., Marks, I.M., Baer, L., Kobak, K.A., et al. (2002). Behavior therapy for obsessive-compulsive disorder guided by a computer or by a clinician compared with relaxation as a control. *Journal of Clinical Psychiatry, 63(2)*: 138–145.

57. Greist, J. (1992). An integrated approach to treatment of obsessive-compulsive disorder. *Journal of Clinical Psychiatry, 53(4)*, 38-41.

58. Mataix-Cols, D., Marks, I.M., Greist, J.H., Kobak, K.A., Baer, L. (2002). Obsessive compulsive symptom dimensions as predictors of compliance with and response to behavior therapy: Results from a controlled trial. *Psychotherapy and Psychosomatics, 71(5)*: 255–262.

59. Beech, H.R. and Vaughn, M. (1978). *Behavioral treatment of obsessive states.* New York: Wiley.

60. Cooper, J.E., Gelder, M.G., and Marks, I.M. (1965). Results of behavior therapy in 77 psychiatric patients. *British Medical Journal, 1*, 1222-1225.

61. Greist, J.H. (1990). Treatment of obsessive-compulsive disorder: Psychotherapies, drugs, and other somatic treatment. *Journal of Clinical Psychiatry, 51*, 44-50.

62. Abramowitz, J.S. (1997). Effectiveness of psychological and pharmacological treatments for obsessive-compulsive disorder: A quantitative review. *Journal of Consulting and Clinical Psychology, 65*, 44-52.

63. van Balkom, A.J.M., van Oppen, P., Vermeulen, A.W.A., van Dyck, R., Nauta, M.C.E., and Vorst, H.C.M. (1994). A meta-analysis on the treatment of obsessive-compulsive disorder: A comparison of antidepressants, behavior, and cognitive therapy. *Clinical Psychology Review, 14,* 359-381.

64. Franklin, M.E., Abramowitz, J.S., Kozak, M.J., Levitt, J.T., and Foa, E.B. (2000). Effectiveness of exposure and ritual prevention for obsessive compulsive disorder: Randomized compared with non-randomized samples. *Journal of Consulting and Clinical Psychology, 68(4),* 594-602.

65. Fritzler, B.K., Hecker, J.E., and Losee, M.C. (1997). Self-directed treatment with minimal therapist contact: Preliminary findings for Obsessive Compulsive Disorder. *Behaviour Research and Therapy, 35,* 627-631.

66. VanDyke, M.M., Pollard, C.A. (2005). Treatment of refractory obsessive-compulsive disorder: The St. Louis Model. *Cognitive and Behavioral Practice, 12*: 30–39.

67. Abramowitz, J.S., Foa, E.B., Franklin, M.E. (2003). Exposure and ritual prevention for obsessive-compulsive disorder: Effects of intensive versus twice-weekly sessions. *Journal of Consulting & Clinical Psychology, 71(2)*: 394–398.

68. Hodgson, R.J., Rachman, S., and Marks, I.M. (1972). The treatment of chronic obsessive-compulsive neurosis: Follow-up and further findings. *Behaviour Research and Therapy, 10,* 181-189.

69. Freeston, M.H., Ladouceur, R., Gagnon, F., Thibodeau, N., Rheaume, J., Letarte, H., and Bujold, A. (1997). Cognitive-behavioral treatment of obsessive thoughts: A controlled study. *Journal of Consulting and Clinical Psychology, 65(3)*, 405-413.

70. Obsessive Compulsive Cognitions Working Group. (1997). Cognitive assessment of obsessive-compulsive disorder. *Behaviour Research and Therapy, 35,* 667-681.

71. Salkovskis, P.M. (1985). Obsessional compulsive problems: A cognitive behavioral analysis. *Behaviour Research and Therapy, 23,* 571-583.

72. Rachman, S., Thordarson, D., Shafran, R., and Woody, S. (1995). Perceived responsibility: Structure and significance. *Behaviour Research and Therapy, 33,* 779-784.

73. Freeston, M., Rh'eume, J., and Ladouceur, R. (1996). Correcting faulty appraisals of obsessional thoughts. *Behaviour Research and Therapy, 34,* 433-446.

74. Libby, S., Reynolds, S., Derisley, J., Clark, S. (2004). Cognitive appraisals in young people with obsessive-compulsive disorder. *Journal of Child Psychology & Psychiatry, 45(6)*: 1076–1084.

75. Ellis, A. (1962). *Reason and emotion in psychotherapy.* New York: Lyle-Stuart.

76. Frost, R.O. (2005). Cognitive-behavioral therapy for OCD. *Behaviour Change, 22(1)*: 50–51.

77. Warren, R. and Zgourides, G. (1991). *Anxiety disorders: A rational emotive perspective.* New York: Pergamon.

78. Steketee, G., and Frost, R.O. (in press). Cognitive theory and treatment of obsessive-compulsive disorder. In M.A. Jenike, L. Baer, and W.E. Minichiello (Eds.), *Obsessive-compulsive disorders: Practical management* (pp. 368-399). St. Louis: Mosby.

79. van Oppen, P., and Arntz, A. (1994). Cognitive therapy for obsessive-compulsive disorder. *Behaviour Research and Therapy, 32,* 79-87.

80. James, I.A., and Blackburn, I. (1995). Cognitive therapy with obsessive-compulsive disorder. *British Journal of Psychiatry, 166,* 444-450.

81. Emmelkamp, P.M.G., Visser, S., and Hoekstra, R.J. (1988). Cognitive therapy vs exposure in vivo in the treatment of obsessive-compulsives. *Cognitive Therapy and Research, 12,* 103-114.

82. Krochmalik, A., Jones, M.K., Menzies, R.G., Kirkby, K. (2004). The superiority of danger ideation reduction therapy (DIRT) over exposure and response prevention (ERP) in treating compulsive washing. *Behavior Change, 21(4)*: 251–268.

83. Emmelkamp, P.M.G. and Beens, H. (1991). Cognitive therapy with obsessive-compulsive disorder: A comparative evaluation. *Behaviour Research and Therapy, 29,* 293-300.

84. van Oppen, P., de Haan, E., van Balkom, A.J.L.M., Spinohoven, P., Hoogduin, K., and van Dyck, R. (1995). Cognitive therapy and exposure in vivo in the treatment of obsessive compulsive disorder. *Behaviour Research and Therapy, 33,* 379-390.

85. Cottraux, J., Note, I., Yao, S.N., LaFont, S., Note, B., Mollard, E., Bouvard, M., Sauteraud, A., Bourgeois, M., and Dartigues, J-F. (2001). A randomized controlled trial of cognitive therapy versus intensive behavior therapy in obsessive compulsive disorder. *Psychotherapy and Psychosomatics, 70(6)*, 288-297.

86. Sifneos, P.E. (1985). Short-term dynamic psychotherapy for patients suffering from an obsessive-compulsive disorder. In Mavissakalian, M., Turner, S.M., and Michelson, L. (Eds.) *Obsessive-compulsive disorder: Psychological and pharmacological treatment.* New York, NY: Plenum Press.

87. Boyarsky, B.K., Perone, L.A., Lee, N.C., and Goodman, W.K. (1991). Current treatment approaches to obsessive-compulsive disorder. *Archives of Psychiatric Nursing, 5*, 299-306.

88. Kobak, K.A., Rock, A.L., and Greist, J.H. (1995). Group behavior therapy for obsessive- compulsive disorder. *The Journal for Specialists in Group Work, 20*, 26-32.

89. Fals-Stewart, W., and Lucente, S. (1994). Behavior group therapy with obsessive-compulsives: An overview. *International Journal of Group Psychotherapy, 44*, 35-51.

90. Black, D.W., and Blum, N.S. (1992). Obsessive-compulsive disorder support groups: The Iowa model. *Comprehensive Psychiatry, 33*, 65-71.

91. Tynes, L.L., Salins, C., Skiba, W., and Winstead, D.K. (1992). A psychoeducational and support group for obsessive-compulsive disorder patients and their significant others. *Comprehensive Psychiatry, 33*, 197-201.

92. Van Noppen, B., Steketee, G., McCorkle, B.H., and Pato, M. (1997). Group and multifamily behavioral treatment for obsessive compulsive disorder: A pilot study. *Journal of Anxiety Disorders, 11(4)*, 431-446.

93. Steketee, G.S., and White, K. (1990). *When once is not enough: Help for obsessive compulsives.* Oakland, CA: New Harbinger.

94. Baer, L. (1991). *Getting control.* Boston: Little, Brown.

95. Foa, E.B., and Wilson, R. (1991). *Stop obsessing!* New York: Bantam.

96. Espie, C.A. (1986). The group treatment of obsessive compulsive ritualizers: Behavioral management of identified patterns of relapse. *Behavioural Psychotherapy, 14*, 21-33.

97. Krone, K.P., Himle, J.A., and Nesse, R.M. (1991). A standardized behavioral group treatment program for obsessive-compulsive disorder: Preliminary outcomes. *Behaviour Research and Therapy, 29*, 627-631.

98. Fals-Stewart, W., Marks, A.P., and Schafer, J. (1993). A comparison of behavioral group therapy and individual behavior therapy in treating obsessive-compulsive disorder. *The Journal of Nervous and Mental Disease, 181*, 189-193.

99. Himle, J.A., Rassi, S., Haghighatgou, H., Krone, K.P., Nesse, R.M., and Abelson, J. (2001). Group behavioral therapy of obsessive-compulsive disorder: Seven- vs. twelve-week outcomes. *Depression and Anxiety 13(4)*, 161-165.

100. Cordioli, A.V., Heldt, E., Bochi, D.B., Margis, R., et al. (2003). Cognitive-behavioral group therapy in obsessive-compulsive disorder: A randomized clinical trial. *Psychotherapy and Psychosomatics, 72(4)*: 211.

101. Chambless, D.L and Steketee, G. (1999). Expressed emotion and behavior therapy outcome: A prospective study with obsessive compulsive and agoraphobia outpatients. *Journal of Consulting and Clinical Psychology. 67(5)*, 658-665.

102. Waters, T.L., Barrett, P.M. and March, J.S. (2001). Cognitive-behavioral family treatment of childhood obsessive-compulsive disorder: Preliminary findings. *American Journal of Psychotherapy, 55(3)*, 372-387.

103. Freeman, J.B., Garcia, A.M., Fucci, C., Karitani, M., et al. (2003). Family-based treatment of early-onset obsessive-compulsive disorder. *Journal of Child & Adolescent Psychopharmacology, 13(2, Suppl)*: S71–S80.

104. Miguel, E.C., Leckman, J.F., Rauch, S., do Rosario-Campos, M.C., Hounie, A.G., Mercadante, M.T., Chacon, P., Pauls, D.L. (2005). Obsessive-compulsive disorder phenotypes: Implications for genetic studies. *Molecular Psychiatry, 10*: 258–275.

105. Harvard Health Publications, Harvard Medical School (2005). Obsessive-compulsive disorder: Part II. *Harvard Mental Health Letter, 22(5)*: 1–4.

106. Lenane, M., Swedo, S., and Leonard, H. (1990). Psychiatric disorders in first degree relatives of children and adolescents with OCD. *Journal of American Academy of Child and Adolescent Psychiatry, 29*, 407-412.

107. Rasmussen, S. (1993). Genetic studies of OCD. *Annals of Clinical Psychiatry, 5*, 241-248.

108. Pauls, D., Alsbrook, J., Goodman, W., Rasmussen, S., and Leckman, J. (1995). A family study of obsessive-compulsive disorder. *American Journal of Psychiatry, 152*, 76-84.

109. Gerald, N., Samuels, J., Riddle, M., Bienvenu III, O.J., Liang, K-Y., LaBuda, M., Walkup, J., Grados, M., and Hoehn-Saric, R. (2000). A family study of obsessive-compulsive disorder. *Archives of General Psychiatry, 57*, 358-363.

110. Billett, E., Richter, M., and Kennedy, J. (1998). Genetics of OCD. In R. Swinson, M. Antony, S. Rachman and M. Richter (Eds.), *OCD: Theory, research, and treatment* (pp. 181-206). New York: The Guilford Press.

111. Antony, M., Downie, F., and Swinson, R. (1998). Diagnostic issues and epidemiology in OCD. In R. Swinson, M. Antony, S. Rachman and M. Richter (Eds.) *OCD: Theory, research, and treatment* (pp. 3-32). New York: The Guilford Press.

112. Pigott, T., L'Heureux, F., Dubbert, B., Bernstein, S., and Murphy, D. (1994). Obsessive-compulsive disorder: Comorbid conditions, *Journal of Clinical Psychiatry, 55(10)*, 15-27.

113. Rasmussen, S. and Eisen, J. (1992). The epidemiology and clinical features of obsessive-compulsive disorder. *Psychiatric Clinics of North America, 15(4)*, 743-758.

114. Crino, R. and Andrews, G. (1996). OCD and Axis I comorbidity, *Journal of Anxiety Disorders, 10*, 37-46.

115. Chen, Y. and Dilsaver, S. (1995). Comorbidity for obsessive-compulsive disorder in bipolar and unipolar disorders. *Psychiatry Research, 59(1-2)*, 57-64.

116. Leonard, H., Lenane, M., Swedo, S., Rettew, D., Gershon, E., and Rapaport, J. (1992). Tics and Tourette's syndrome: A two- to seven-year follow-up of 54 OCD children, *American Journal of Psychiatry, 149*, 1244-1251.

117. Pauls, D.L., Pakstis, A.J., Kurlan, R., Kidd, K.K., Leckman, J.F., Cohen, D.J., Kidd, J.R., Como, P., and Sparkes, R. (1990). Segregation and linkage analyses of Tourette's syndrome and related disorders. *Journal of American Academy of Child and Adolescent Psychiatry, 29(2)*, 195-203.

118. Goodman, W., McDougle, C., Price, L., Riddle, M., Pauls, D., and Leckman, J. (1990). Beyond the serotonin hypothesis: A role for dopamine in some forms of obsessive-compulsive disorder? *Journal of Clinical Psychiatry, 51(8)*, 36-43.

119. Baxter, L. and Guze, B. (1992). Neuroimaging. In R. Kurlan (Ed.), *Handbook of Tourette's syndrome and related tic and behavioral disorders* (pp. 289-304). New York: Dekker.

120. Chase, T., Foster, N., Fenio, P., Brooks, R., Monsi, L., Kessler, R., and Di Chiro, G. (1984). Gilles de la Tourette syndrome: Studies with fluorine 18 labeled fluorodeoxyglucose positron emission tomographic methods. *Annals of Neurology, 15*, 175.

121. Saxena, S., Bota, R.G., and Brody, A.L. (2001). Brain-behavior relationships in obsessive-compulsive disorder. *Seminars in Clinical Neuropsychiatry, 6(2)*, 82-101.

122. Brody, A. and Saxena, S. (1996). Brain imaging in OCD: Evidence for the involvement of frontal-subcortical circuitry in the mediation of symptomatology. *CNS Spectrums, 1*, 27-41.

123. Otto, M.W. (1992). Normal and abnormal information processing: A neuropsychological perspective on obsessive compulsive disorder. *Psychiatric Clinics of North America, 15(4)*, 825-48.

124. Rosenberg, D., Dick, E., O'Hearn, K., and Sweeney, J. (1997). Response-inhibition deficits in obsessive-compulsive disorder: An indicator of dysfunction in frontostriatal circuits. *Journal of Psychiatry and Neurosciences, 22(1)*, 29-38.

125. Stahl, S. (1988). Basal ganglia neuropharmacology and obsessive-compulsive disorder: The obsessive-compulsive disorder hypothesis of basal ganglion dysfunction. *Psychopharmacology Bulletin, 24(3)*, 370-374.

126. Hugo, F., van Heerden, B., Zungu-Dirwayi, N., and Stein, D.J. (1999). Functional brain imaging in obsessive-compulsive disorder secondary to neurological lesions. *Depression and Anxiety, 10(3)*, 129-136.

127. Pitman, R., Green, R., Jenike, M., and Mesulam, M. (1987). Animal models of OCD. *American Journal of Psychiatry, 143*, 1166-1171.

128. Rapaport, J. (1992). An animal model of obsessive-compulsive disorder. *Archives of General Psychiatry, 49*, 517-521.

129. Yadin, E., Friedman, E., and Bridger, W.H. (1991). Spontaneous alternation behavior: An animal model for obsessive-compulsive disorder? *Pharmacology and Biochemistry of Behavior, 40(2)*, 311-5.

130. Greenberg, B.D., Ziemann, U., Cora-Locatelli, G., Harmon, A., Murphy, D.L., Keel, J.C., and Wassermann, E.M. (2000). Altered cortical excitability in obsessive-compulsive disorder. *Neurology, 54(1)*, 142-147.

131. Muller, N., Putz, A., Kathmann, N., Lehle, R., Gunther, W., and Straube, A. (1997). Characteristics of obsessive-compulsive symptoms in Tourette's syndrome, obsessive-compulsive disorder, and Parkinson's disease. *Psychiatry Research, 70(2)*, 105-114.

132. van den Heuvel, O.A., Veltman, D.J., Groenewegen, H.J., Dolan, R.J., et al. (2004). Amygdala activity in obsessive-compulsive disorder with contamination fear: A study with oxygen-15 water positron emission tomography. *Psychiatry Research: Neuroimaging, 132(3)*: 225–237.

133. Cannistraro, P.A., Wright, C.I., Wedig, M.M., Martis, B., et al. (2004). Amygdala responses to human faces in obsessive-compulsive disorder. *Biological Psychiatry, 56(12)*: 916–920.

134. Sydenham's Chorea (Chorea Minor; Rheumatic Chorea; St. Vitus' Dance). (1999). *The Merck Manual of Diagnosis and Therapy*, 17.

135. Swedo, S., Kilpatrick, K., Schapiro, M., Leonard, H., Cheslow, D., and Rapaport, J. (1991). Antineuronal antibodies in Sydenham's chorea and obsessive-compulsive disorder. *Pediatric Research, 29*, 364A.

136. Swedo, S., Rapaport, J., Cheslow, D., Leonard, H., Ayoub, E., Hosier, D., and Wald, E. (1989). High prevalence of obsessive-compulsive disorder symptoms in patients with Sydenham's chorea. *American Journal of Psychiatry, 146*, 246-249.

137. Kiessling, L.S., Marcotte, A.C., and Culpepper, L. (1994). Antineuronal antibodies: Tics and obsessive-compulsive symptoms. *Journal of Developmental and Behavioral Pediatrics, 15(6)*, 421-5.

138. Arnold, P.D. and Richter, M.A. (2001). Is obsessive-compulsive disorder an autoimmune disease? *Canadian Medical Association Journal, 165(10)*, 1353-1358.

139. Murphy, M.L. and Pichichero, M.E. (2002). Prospective identification and treatment of children with pediatric autoimmune neuropsychiatric disorder associated with group a streptococcal infection (PANDAS). *Archives of Pediatric Adolescent Medicine, 156*, 356-361.

140. Asbahr, F.R., Negrao, A.B., Gentil, V., Zanetta, D.M.T., da Paz, J.A., Marques-Dias, M.J., and Kiss, M.H. (1998). Obsessive-compulsive and related symptoms in children and adolescents with rheumatic fever with and without chorea: A prospective 6-month study. *American Journal of Psychiatry, 155(8)*, 1122-1124

141. Giedd, J.N., Rapoport, J.L., Garvey, M.A., Perlmutter, S., and Swedo, S.E. (2000). MRI assessment of children with obsessive-compulsive disorder or tics associated with streptococcoal infection. *American Journal of Psychiatry, 157(2)*, 281-283.

142. Peterson, B.S., Leckman, J.T., Tucker, D., Scahill, L., Staib, L., Zhang, H., King, R., Cohen, D.J., Gore, J.C., and Lombroso, P. (2000). Preliminary findings of antistreptococcal antibody titers and basal ganglia volumes in tic, obsessive-compulsive, and attention deficit/hyperactivity disorders. *Archives of General Psychiatry, 57(4)*, 364-372.

143. Leonard, H. and Swedo, S.E. (2001). Paediatric autoimmune neuropsychiatric disorders associated with streptococcal infection (PANDAS). *International Journal of Neuropsychopharmacology, 4(2)*, 191-198.

144. Swedo, S.E., Leonard, H.L., Garvey, M., Mittleman, B., Allen, A.J., Perlmutter, S., Lougee, L., Dow, S., Zamkoff, J., and Dubbert, B.K. (1998). Pediatric autoimmune neuropsychiatric disorders associated with streptococcal infections: Clinical description of the first 50 cases. *American Journal of Psychiatry, 155(2)*, 264-271.

145. Baxter, L., Schwatrz, J., Guze, B., Bergman, K., and Szuba, M. (1990). Neuroimaging in OCD: Seeking the mediating neuroanatomy. In M. Jenike, L. Baer, and W. Minichiello (Eds.) *OCDs: Theory and management* (pp. 167-188). St. Louis: Mosby YearBook.

146. Rauch, S. and Savage, C. (1997). Neuroimaging and neuropsychology of the striatum: Bridging basic science and clinical practice. *Psychiatric Clinics of North America, 20(4)*, 741-68.

147. Jenike, M., Breiter, H., Baer, L., Kennedy, D., Savage, C., Olivares, M., O'Sullivan, R., Shera, D., Rauch, S., Kenthen, N., Rosen, B., Caviness, V., and Filipek, P. (1996). Cerebral structural abnormalities in OCD. *Archives of General Psychiatry, 53*, 625-632.

148. Kang, D., Kim, J., Choi, J., Kim, Y., et al. (2004). Volumetric investigation of the frontal-subcortical circuitry in patients with obsessive-compulsive disorder. *Journal of Neuropsychiatry & Clinical Neurosciences, 16(3)*: 342–349.

149. Whiteside, S.P., Port, J.D., Abramowitz, J.S. (2003). A meta-analysis of functional neuroimaging in obsessive-compulsive disorder. *Psychiatry Research: Neuroimaging, 132*: 69–79.

150. Schienle, A., Schäfer, A., Stark, R., Walker, B., Vaitl, D. (2005). Neural responses of OCD patients towards disorder-relevant, generally disgust-inducing and fear-inducing pictures. *International Journal of Psychophysiology, 57(1)*: 69–77.

151. Abbruzzese, M., Ferri, S., and Scarone, S. (1995). Wisconsin Card Sorting Test performance in obsessive-compulsive disorder: No evidence for involvement of dorsolateral prefrontal cortex. *Psychiatry Research, 58(1)*, 37-43.

152. Cumming, S., Hay, P., Lee, T., and Sachdev, P. (1995). Neuropsychological outcome from psychosurgery for obsessive-compulsive disorder. *Australia and New Zealand Journal of Psychiatry, 29(2)*, 293-8.

153. Azmitia, E. and Whitaker-Azmitia, P. (1991). Awakening the sleeping giant: Anatomy and plasticity of the brain serotonergic system. *Journal of Clinical Psychiatry, 52*, 4-16.

154. Baumgarten, H. and Grozdanovic, Z. (1995). Psychopharmacology of central serotonergic systems. *Pharmacopsychiatry, 28*, 73-9.

155. Barr, L., Goodman, W., Price, L., McDougle, C., and Charney, D. (1992). The serotonin hypothesis of obsessive-compulsive disorder: Implications of pharmacologic challenge studies. *Journal of Clinical Psychiatry, 53(4)*, 17-28.

156. Jefferson, J.W., Altemus, M., Jenike, M. A., Pigott, T.A., Stein, D. J., and Greist, J.H. (1995). Algorithm for the treatment of obsessive-compulsive disorder (OCD). *Psychopharmacology Bulletin, 31(3)*, 487-490.

157. Murphy, D.L. and Pigott, T.A. (1990). A comparative examination of a role for serotonin in obsessive-compulsive disorder, panic disorder, and anxiety. *Journal of Clinical Psychiatry, 51*.

158. Pigott, T. (1996). OCD: Where the serotonin-selectivity story begins. *Journal of Clinical Psychiatry, 57(6)*, 11-20.

159. Zohar, J. and Insel, T. (1987). Obsessive-compulsive disorder: Psychobiological approaches to diagnosis, treatment, and pathophysiology. *Biological Psychiatry, 22*, 667-687.

160. Hollander, E., DeCaria, C., Nitescu, A., Gully, R., Suckow, R., Cooper, T., Gorman, J., Klein, D., and Liebowitz, M. (1992). Serotonergic function in obsessive-compulsive disorder: Behavioral and neuroendocrine responses to oral m-CPP and fenfluramine in patients and healthy volunteers. *Archives of General Psychiatry, 49*, 21-28.

161. Barr, L., Goodman, W., McDougle, C., and Delgado, P. (1994). Tryptophan depletion in patients with obsessive-compulsive disorder who respond to serotonin reuptake inhibitors. *Archives of General Psychiatry, 51(4)*, 309-317.

162. Benkelfat, C., Murphy, D., Zohar, J., Hill, J., Grover, G., and Insel, T. (1989). Clomipramine in obsessive-compulsive disorder: Further evidence for a serotonergic mechanism of action. *Archives of General Psychiatry, 46*, 23-28.

163. Hollander, E., DeCaria, C., Nitescu, A., Gorman, J., Klein, D., and Liebowitz, M. (1991). Noradrenergic function in obsessive-compulsive disorder: Behavioral and neuroendocrine responses to clonidine and comparison to healthy controls. *Psychiatry Research, 137*, 161-177.

164. Marazziti, D., Hollander, E., Lensi, P., Ravagli, S., and Cassano, G. (1992). Peripheral markers of serotonin and dopamine function in obsessive-compulsive disorder. *Psychiatry Research, 42(1)*, 41-51.

165. Greist, J., Jefferson, J., Koback, K., Katzelnick, D., and Serlin, R. (1995). Efficacy and tolerability of serotonin transport inhibitors in obsessive-compulsive disorder: A meta-analysis. *Archives of General Psychiatry, 52*, 53-60.

166. Pigott, T. and Seay, S. (1997). Pharmacotherapy of OCD. *International Review of Psychiatry, 9(1)*, 133-147.

167. Dougherty, D.D., Rauch, S.L., Jenike, M.A. (2004). Pharmacotherapy for obsessive-compulsive disorder. *Journal of Clinical Psychology, 60(11)*: 1195–1202.

168. Fineberg, N.A., Gale, T.M. (2005). Evidence-based pharmacotherapy of obsessive-compulsive disorder. *International Journal of Neuropsychopharmacology, 8*: 107–129.

169. Geller, D.A., Biederman, J., Stewart, S.E., Mullin, B., et al. (2003). Which SSRI? A meta-analysis of pharmacotherapy trials in pediatric obsessive-compulsive disorder. *The American Journal of Psychiatry, 160(11)*: 1919.

170. Preskorn, S. (1996). *Clinical pharmacology of selective serotonin reuptake inhibitors.* (1st ed.). Caddo, OK: Professional Communications, Inc.

171. Keuthen, N., Cyr, P., Ricciardi, J., and Minichiello, W. (1994). Medication withdrawal symptoms in obsessive-compulsive disorder patients treated with paroxetine. *Journal of Clinical Psychopharmacology, 14(3)*, 206-207.

172. Frost, L. and Sal, S. (1995). Shock-like sensations after discontinuation of selective serotonin reuptake inhibitors. *American Journal of Psychiatry, 152(5)*, 810.

173. Celexa Prescribing Information (2002). www.celexa.com/prescribing_information/prescribing_information.asp, New York, NY: Forest Pharameuticals, Inc.

174. Montgomery, S.A., Kasper, S., Stein, D.J., Bang, H.K., and Lemming, O.M. (2001). Citalopram 20 mg, 40 mg and 50 mg are all effective and well tolerated compared with placebo in obsessive-compulsive disorder. *International Journal of Clinical Psychopharmacology, 16(2)*, 75-86.

175. Thomsen, P.H., Ebbesen, C., and Persson, C. (2001). Long-term experience with citalopram in the treatment of adolescent OCD. *Journal of the American Academy of Child and Adolescent Psychiatry, 40(8)*, 895-902.

176. Marazziti, D., Dell'Osso, L., Gemignani, A., Presta, S., Nasso, E.D., Pfanner, C., and Cassano, G.B. (2001). Citalopram in refractory obsessive-compulsive disorder: An open study. *International Journal of Clinical Psychopharmacology, 16(4)*, 215-219.

177. Mukaddes, N.M., Abali, O., Kaynak, N. (2003). Citalopram treatment of children and adolescents with obsessive-compulsive disorder: A preliminary report. *Psychiatry and Clinical Neurosciences, 57(4)*: 405–408.

178. Pallanti, S., Quercioli, L., Koran, L.M. (2002). Citalopram intravenous infusion in resistant obsessive-compulsive disorder: An open trial. *Journal of Clinical Psychiatry, 63(9)*: 796–801.

179. Pallanti, S., Quercioli, L., Bruscoli, M. (2004). Response acceleration with mirtazapine augmentation of citalopram in obsessive-compulsive disorder patients without comorbid depression: A pilot study. *Journal of Clinical Psychiatry, 65(10)*: 1394–1399.

180. Tollefson, G., Rampey, A., Potvin, J., and Fenike, M. (1994). A multicenter investigation of fixed-dose fluoxetine in the treatment of obsessive-compulsive disorder. *Archives of General Psychiatry, 51(7)*, 559-567.

181. Geller, D.A. (2001). Fluoxetine treatment for obsessive-compulsive disorder in children and adolescents: A placebo-controlled clinical trial. *Journal of the American Academy of Child and Adolescent Psychiatry, 40(7)*, 773-779.

182. Prozac Product/Prescribing Information (2001) www.prozac.com/HowProzacCanHelp/PrescriptionInformation.jsp, Eli Lilly and Company.

183. Kronig, M.H., Apter, J., Asnis, G., Bystritsky, A., Curtis, G., Ferguson, J., Landbloom, R., Munjack, D., Riesenberg, R., Robinson, D., Roy-Byrne, P., Phillips, K., and DuPont, I.J. (1999). Placebo-controlled, multicenter study of sertraline treatment for obsessive-compulsive disorder. *Journal of Clinical Psychopharmacology, 19(2)*, 172-176.

184. Cook, E.H., Wagner, K.D., March, J.S., Biederman, J., Landau, P., Wolkow, R., and Messig, M. (2001). Long-term sertraline treatment of children and adolescents with obsessive-compulsive disorder. *Journal of the American Academy of Child and Adolescent Psychiatry, 40(10)*, 1175-1181.

185. Zoloft prescribing information (2001) www.zoloft.com, Pfizer, Inc.

186. Koran, L.M., Hackett, E., Rubin, A., Wolkow, R., Robinson, D. (2002). Efficacy of sertraline in the long-term treatment of obsessive-compulsive disorder. *The American Journal of Psychiatry, 159(1)*: 88–95.

187. Wagner, K.D., Cook, E.H., Chung, H., Messig, M. (2003). Remission status after long-term sertraline treatment of pediatric obsessive-compulsive disorder. *Journal of Child & Adolescent Psychopharmacology, 13(2 Suppl)*: S53–S60.

188. Wheadon, D., Bushnell, W., and Steiner, M. (1993). "A fixed-dose comparison of 20, 40, or 60 mg. paroxetine to placebo in the treatment of obsessive-compulsive disorder." Paper presented at the American College of Neuropsychopharmacology (ACNP) Annual Meeting, San Juan, PR.

189. Rosenberg, D.R., Stewart, C.M., Fitzgerald, K.D., Tawile, V., and Carroll, E. (1999). Paroxetine open-label treatment of pediatric outpatients with obsessive-compulsive disorder. *Journal of the American Academy of Child and Adolescent Psychiatry, 38(9)*, 1180-1185.

190. Paxil Prescribing Information (2002), Philadelphia, PA: GlaxoSmithKline.

191. Hollander, E., Allen, A., Steiner, M., Wheadon, D.E., et al. (2003). Acute and long-term treatment and prevention of relapse of obsessive-compulsive disorder with paroxetine. *Journal of Clinical Psychiatry, 64(9)*: 1113–1121.

192. Tenney, N.H., Denys, D.A.J.P., van Megen, H.J.G.M., Glas, G., Westenberg, H.G.M. (2003). Effect of a pharmacological intervention on quality of life in patients with obsessive-compulsive disorder. *International Clinical Psychopharmacology, 18(1)*: 29–33.

193. Geller, D.A., Biederman, J., Stewart, S.E., Mullin, B. (2003). Impact of comorbidity on treatment response to paroxetine in pediatric obsessive-compulsive disorder: Is the use of exclusion criteria empirically supported in randomized clinical trials? *Journal of Child & Adolescent Psychopharmacology, 13(2, Suppl)*: S19–S29.

194. Geller, D.A., Wagner, K.D., Emslie, G., Murphy, T., et al. (2004). Paroxetine treatment in children and adolescents with obsessive-compulsive disorder: A randomized, multicenter, double-blind, placebo-controlled trial. *Journal of the American Academy of Child & Adolescent Psychiatry, 43(11)*: 1387–1396.

195.. Riddle, M.A., Reeve, E.A., Yaryura-Tobias, J.A., Yang, H.M., Claghorn, J.L., Gaffney, G., Greist, J.H., Holland, D., McConville, B.J., Pigott, T., and Walkup, J.T. (2001). Fluoxamine for children and adolescents with obsessive-compulsive disorder: A randomized, controlled, multicenter trial. *Journal of the American Academy of Child and Adolescent Psychiatry, 40(2)*, 222-229.

196. Hollander, E., Koran, L.M., Goodman, W.K., Greist, J.H., et al. (2003). A double-blind, placebo-controlled study of the efficacy and safety of controlled-release fluvoxamine in patients with obsessive-compulsive disorder. *Journal of Clinical Psychiatry, 64(6)*: 640–647.

197. Luvox Prescribing Information (2000), Marietta, GA: Solvay Pharmaceuticals, Inc.

198. DeVane, C. (1992). Pharmacokinetics of the selective serotonin reuptake inhibitors. *Journal of Clinical Psychiatry, 53(2)*, 13-20.

199. Saxena, S., Brody, A.L., Ho, M.L., Zohrabi, N., et al. (2003). Differential brain metabolic predictors of response to paroxetine in obsessive-compulsive disorder versus major depression. *The American Journal of Psychiatry, 160(3)*: 522–533.

200. Goodman, W., McDougle, C., Barr, L., and Price, L. (1993). Biological approaches to the treatment-refractory patient. *1st International OCD Conference Abstracts, Isle of Capri (Italy)*, 139-140.

201. Jenike, M. and Raush, S. (1994). Managing the patient with treatment-resistant obsessive-compulsive disorder: Current strategies. *Journal of Clinical Psychiatry, 55*, 11-17.

202. Rasmussen, S., Eisen, J., and Pato, M. (1993). Current issues in the pharmacological management of obsessive-compulsive disorder. *Journal of Clinical Psychiatry, 54(6)*, 4-9.

203. Mundo, E., Bareggi, S., Pirola, R., Bellodi, L., and Smeraldi, E. (1997). Long-term pharmacotherapy of obsessive-compulsive disorder: A double-blind controlled study. *Journal of Clinical Psychopharmacology, 17(1)*, 4-10.

204. Pato, M., Hill, J., and Murphy, D. (1990). A clomipramine dosage reduction study in the course of long-term treatment of OCD patients. *Psychopharmacology Bulletin, 26*, 211-214.

205. Pato, M., Zohar-Kadouch, R., Zohar, J., and Murphy, D. (1988). Return of symptoms after discontinuation of clomipramine in patients with obsessive-compulsive disorder. *American Journal of Psychiatry, 145*, 1521-1525.

206. Leonard, H., Swedo, S., Lenane, M., Rettew, D., Cheslow, D., Hamburger, S., and Rapaport, J. (1991). A double-blind desipramine substitution during long-term clomipramine treatment in children and adolescents with obsessive-compulsive disorder. *Archives of General Psychiatry, 48*, 922-927.

207. Steiner, M., Bushnell, W., Gergel, I., and Wheadon, D. (1995). "Long-term treatment and prevention of relapse of OCD with paroxetine." Paper presented at the American Psychiatric Association Annual Meeting, Miami, FL, May 9-12.

208. Koran, L.M., Hackett, E., Rubin, A., Wolkow, R., and Robinson, D. (2002). Efficacy of sertraline in the long-term treatment of obsessive-compulsive disorder. *American Journal of psychiatry, 159(1)*, 88-95.

209. Romano, S., Goodman, W., Tamura, R., and Gonzales, J. (2001). Long-term treatment of obsessive-compulsive disorder after an acute response: a comparison of fluoxetine versus placebo. *Journal of Clinical Psychopharmacology*, 21(1), 46-52.

210. Atmaca, M., Kuloglu, M., Tezcan, E., Gecici, O. (2002). Quetiapine augmentation in patients with treatment resistant obsessive-compulsive disorder: A single-blind, placebo study. *International Clinical Psychopharmacology, 17(3)*: 115–119.

211. Denys, D., de Geus, F., van Megen, H.J.G.M., Westenberg, H.G.M. (2004). A double-blind, randomized, placebo-controlled trial of quetiapine addition in pateints with obsessive-compulsive refractory to serotonin reuptake inhibitors. *Journal of Clinical Psychiatry, 65(8)*: 1040–1048.

212. Fineberg, N.A., Sivakumaran, T., Roberts, A., Gale, T. (2005). Adding quetiapine to SRI in treatment-resistant obsessive-compulsive disorder: A randomized controlled treatment study. *International Clinical Psychopharmacolgy, 20(4)*: 223–226.

213. Sareen, J., Kirshner, A., Lander, M., Kjernisted, K.D., Eleff, M.K., Reiss, J.P. (2004). Do antipsychotics ameliorate or exacerbate obsessive compulsive disorder symptoms? A systematic review. *Journal of Affective Disorders, 82(2)*: 167–174.

214. Keuneman, R.J., Pokos, V., Weerasundera, R., Castle, D.J. (2005). Antipsychotic treatment in obsessive-compulsive disorder: A literature review. *Australian & New Zealand Journal of Psychiatry, 39(5)*: 336–343.

215. McDougle, C.J., Epperson, N., Pelton, G.H., Wasylink, S., and Price, L.H. et al (2000). A double-blind, placebo-controlled study of risperidone addition in serotonin reuptake inhibitor-refractory, obsessive-compulsive disorder. *Archives of General Psychiatry, 57*, 794-801.

216. McDougle, C., Goodman, W., Leckman, J., and Lee, N. (1994). Haloperidol addition in fluvoxamine-refractory obsessive-compulsive disorder: A double-blind, placebo-controlled study in patients with and without tics. *Archives of General Psychiatry, 51(4)*, 302-308.

217. McDougle, C. (1994). Risperidone augmentation for refractory OCD. An open study. *Journal of Clinical Psychiatry*.

218. McDougle, C.J., Fleischmann, R.L., Epperson, C.N., Wasylink, S., Leckman, J.F., and Price, L.H. (1995). Risperidone addition in fluvoxamine-refractory obsessive-compulsive disorder: Three cases. *Journal of Clinical Psychiatry, 56(11)*, 526-8.

219. Saxena, S., Wang, D., Bystritsky, A., and Baxter, L.R., Jr. (1996). Risperidone augmentation of SRI treatment for refractory obsessive-compulsive disorder. *Journal of Clinical Psychiatry, 57(7)*, 303-6.

220. Crockett, B.A., Churchill, E., Davidson, J.R. (2004). A double-blind combination study of clonazepam with sertraline in obsessive-compulsive disorder. *Annals of Clinical Psychiatry, 16(3)*: 127–132.

221. Prasad, A. (1985). Efficacy of trazodone as an antiobsessional agent. *Pharmacology and Biochemistry of Behavior, 22*, 347-348.

222. Pigott, T.A., L'Heureux, F., Rubenstein, C.S., Bernstein, S.E., Hill, J.L., and Murphy, D.L. (1992). A double-blind, placebo controlled study of trazodone in patients with obsessive-compulsive disorder. *Journal of Clinical Psychopharmacology, 12(3)*, 156-162.

223. Koran, L.M., Gamel, N.N., Choung, H.W., Smith, E.H., Aboujaoude, E.N. (2005). Mirtazapine for obsessive-compulsive disorder: An open trial followed by double-blind discontinuation. *Journal of Clinical Psychiatry, 66(4)*: 515–520.

224. Rauch, S., O'Sullivan, R., and Jenike, M. (1996). Open treatment of obsessive-compulsive disorder with venlafaxine: A series of ten cases. *Journal of Clinical Psychopharmacology, 16(1)*, 81-84.

225. Yayura-Tobias, J. (1996). Venlafaxine in OCD. *Psychopharmacology Bulletin*.

226. Albert, U., Aguglia, E., Maina, G., Bogetto, F. (2002). Venlafaxine versus clomipramine in the treatment of obsessive-compulsive disorder: A preliminary single-blind, 12-week, controlled study. *Journal of Clinical Psychiatry, 63(11)*: 1004–1009.

227. Denys, D., van Megen, H.J.G.M., van der Wee, N., Westenberg, H.G.M. (2004). A double-blind switch study of paroxetine and venlafaxine in obsessive-compulsive disorder. *Journal of Clinical Psychiatry, 65(1)*: 37–43.

228. Denys, D., van der Wee, N., van Megen, H.J.G.M., Westenberg, H.G.M. (2003). A double blind comparison of venlafaxine and paroxetine in obsessive-compulsive disorder. *Journal of Clinical Psychopharmacology, 23(6)*: 568–575.

229. Carrasco, J., Hollander, E., Schneier, F., and Liebowitz, M. (1992). Treatment outcome of OCD with comorbid social phobia. *Journal of Clinical Psychiatry, 53*, 387-391.

230. Jenike, M., Surnam, O., and Cassem, N. (1983). Monoamine oxidase inhibitors in OCD. *Journal of Clinical Psychiatry, 44*, 131-132.

231. Schulman, K., Walker, S., MacKenzie, S., and Knowles, S. (1989). Dietary restrictions, tyramine, and the uses of monoamine oxidase inhibitors. *Journal of Clinical Psychopharmacology, 9*, 397-402.

232. Dougherty, D.D., Baer, L., Cosgrove, G.R., Cassem, E.H., Price, B.H., Nierenberg, A.A., Jenike, M.A., and Rauch, S.C. (2002). Prospective long-term follow-up of 44 patients who received cingulotomy for treatment-refractory obsessive-compulsive disorder. *American Journal of Psychiatry, 159(2)*, 269-275.

233. Baer, L., Rauch, S., Ballantine, T., and Martuza, R. (1995). Cingulotomy for intractable OCD: Prospective long-term follow-up of 18 patients. *Archives of General Psychiatry, 52(5)*, 384-392.

234. Hay, P., Sachdev, P., Cumming, S., Smith, J.S., Lee, T., Kitchener, P., and Matheson, J. (1993). Treatment of obsessive-compulsive disorder by psychosurgery. *Acta Psychiatrica Scandinavia, 87(3)*, 197-207.

235. Mindus, P., Rasmussen, S.A., and Lindquist, C. (1994). Neurosurgical treatment for refractory obsessive-compulsive disorder: Implications for understanding frontal lobe function. *Journal of Neuropsychiatry and Clinical Neurosciences, 6(4)*, 467-77.

236. Rabheru, K. and Persad, E. (1997). A review of continuation and maintenance electroconvulsive therapy. *Canadian Journal of Psychiatry, 42(5)*, 476-84.

237. Casey, D. and Davis, M. (1994). Obsessive-compulsive disorder responsive to electroconvulsive therapy in an elderly woman. *Southern Medical Journal, 87(8)*, 862-4.

238. Nakatani, E., Nakagawa, A., Nakao, T., Yoshizato, C., Nabeyama, M., Kudo, A., Isomura, K., Kato, N., Yoshioka, K., Kawamoto, M. (2005). A randomized controlled trial of Japanese patients with obsessive-compulsive disorder — effectiveness of behavior therapy and fluvoxamine. *Psychotherapy and Psychosomatics, 74(5)*: 269–276.

239. Foa, E.B., Liebowitz, M.R., Kozak, M.J., Davies, S., et al. (2005). Randomized, placebo-controlled trial of exposure and ritual prevention, clomipramine, and their combination in the treatment of obsessive-compulsive disorder. *The American Journal of Psychiatry, 162(1)*: 151–161.

240. Abramowitz, J.S., Whiteside, S.P., Deacon, B.J. (2005). The effectiveness of treatment for pediatric obsessive-compulsive disorder: A meta-analysis. *Behavior Therapy, 36(1)*: 55–63.

241. Fang-Ru, Y., Shuang-Luo, Z., Wen-Feng, L. (2005). Comparative study of solution-focused brief therapy (SFBT) combined with paroxetine in the treatment of obsessive-compulsive disorder. *Chinese Mental Health Journal, 19(4)*: 288–290.

242. Simpson, H.B., Franklin, M.E., Cheng, J., Foa, E.B., Liebowitz, M.R. (2005). Standard criteria for relapse are needed in obsessive-compulsive disorder. *Depression & Anxiety, 21(1)*: 1–8.

243. Kordon, A., Kahl, K.G., Broocks, A., Voderholzer, U., et al. (2005). Clinical outcome in patients with obsessive-compulsive disorder after discontinuation of SRI treatment: Results from a two-year follow-up. *European Archives of Psychiatry & Clinical Neuroscience, 255(1)*: 48–50.

244. Simpson, H.B., Liebowitz, M.R., Foa, E.B., Kozak, M.J., et al. (2004). Post-treatment effects of exposure therapy and clomipramine in obsessive-compulsive disorder. *Depression & Anxiety, 19(4)*: 225–233.

245. Baer, L. (1993). Behavior therapy for obsessive-compulsive disorder in the office-based practice. *Journal of Clinical Psychiatry, 54*, 10-15.

246. Shaomei, L. et al. (2001). Combination of clominpramine with exposure therapy in treatment of obsessive-compulsive disorder. *Chinese Mental Health Journal, 15*(4), 239-240.

247. De Hann, E., Huyser, C., Boer, F. (2005). Obsessive-compulsive disorder in children and adolescents. *Tijdschrift voor Psychiatrie, 47(4)*: 229–238.

248. Pediatric OCD Treatment Study (POTS) Team. (2004). Cognitive-behavior therapy, sertraline, and their combination for children and adolescents with obsessive-compulsive disorder: The Pediatric OCD Treatment Study (POTS) randomized controlled trial. *Journal of the American Medical Association, 292(16):* 1969–1976.

249. O'Connor, K., Todorov, C., Robillard, S., Borgeat, F., and Brault, M. (1999). Cognitive-behaviour therapy and medication in the treatment of obsessive-compulsive disorder: A controlled study. *Canadian Journal of Psychiatry, 44:* 64, 7p, 3 charts.

250. Foa, E.B., Huppert, J.D., Lieberg, S., Langner, R., Kichic, R., Hajcak, G., Salkovskis, P.M. (2002). The obsessive-compulsive inventory: Development and validation of a short version. *Psychological Assessment, 14,* 485–495.

251. Sanavio, E. (1988). Obsessions and compulsions: The Padua Inventory. *Behaviour Research and Therapy, 26,* 169-177.

252. Williams, M.T., Turkheimer, E., Schmidt, K.M., Oltmanns, T.F. (2005). Ethnic identification biases responses to the Padua Inventory for obsessive-compulsive disorder. *Assessement, 12(2):* 174–185.

253. Thordarson, D.S., Radmonsky, A.S., Rachman, S., Shafran, R., et al. (2004). The Vancouver Obsessional Compulsive Inventory (VOCI). *Behaviour Research & Therapy, 42(11):* 1289–1314.

254. First, M.B., Spitzer, R.L., Gibbon, M., and Williams, J.B.W. (1995). *Structured Clinical Interview for DSM-IV Axis I Disorders - Patient Edition (SCID-I/P, Version 2)*, New York: New York State Psychiatric Institute.

255. DiNardo, P. A. and Barlow, D.H. (1998). *Anxiety Disorders Interview Schedule-Revised.* Albany, NY: Graywind.

256. Goodman, W.K., Price, L.H., Rasmussen, S.A., Mazure, C., Fleischmann, R.L., Hill, C.L., Heninger, G.R., and Charney, D.S. (1989). The Yale-Brown Obsessive-Compulsive Scale: I. Development, use, and reliability. *Archives of General Psychiatry, 46,* 1006-1011.

257. Storch, E.A., Murphy, T.K., Gefken, G.R., Soto, O., et al. (2004). Psychometric evaluation of the Children's Yale-Brown Obsessive-Compulsive Scale. *Psychiatry Research, 129(1):* 91–98.

258. Ulloa, R.E., de la Peña, F., Higuera, F., Palacos, L., et al. (2004). Validity and reliability of the Spanish version of Yale-Brown rating scale for children and adolescents. *Actas Españolas de Psiquiatria, 32(4):* 216–221.

Index

A

Addictive disorders 15, 16
Age of onset 2, 11
Amygdala 54, 55
Anafranil® *See* Clomipramine
Antianxiety agents
    Buspirone (BuSpar®) 66, 67
    Clonazepam (Klonopin®) 66, 67, 68
    Oxazepam (Serax®) 67
Antidepressants 57, 59, 61, 63,
    67, 70 *See also* SRIs
    Cyclic antidepressants 67
        Mirtazapine (Remeron®) 63, 67, 68
        Trazodone (Desyrel®) 67
        Venlafaxine (Effexor®) 67, 68
    MAOIs (Monoamine oxidase
      inhibitors) 67
        Phenelzine (Nardil®) 67
        Tranylcypromine (Parnate®) 67
Antimanic agent
    Lithium (Eskalith®) 66
Antipsychotics
    Haloperidol (Haldol®) 66
    Pimozide (Orap®) 66
Anxiety 1
    and assessment 8, 16, 17, 18, 19
    and pharmacotherapy 53, 58, 59, 62, 66, 67
    and psychotherapy 22, 23, 24, 26, 27, 28,
      29, 31, 32, 33, 34, 37, 38, 39, 42, 43, 46
Anxiety disorder(s) 1, 11, 53
Anxiety Disorders Interview
   Schedule (ADIS) 14, 75
Anxiety disorder due to a general
   medical condition 15, 16
Assessment tools 10–15 *See*
   also individual tools
    Behavior assessment 14–15 *See*
     also Behavioral avoidance
     tests (BAT); SUDS
    Clinical interviews 10–13, 14, 75
    Laboratory/physical exam findings 10, 15
    Psychometric assessments 10, 15, 73
    Self-report instruments 10, 13–14, 73–74
    Structured interviews 10,
     13–14, 73, 75–76
Atypical antipsychotics 66
    Olanzapine (Zyprexa®) 66
    Quetiapine (Seroquel®) 66

Risperidone (Risperdal®) 66, 68
Augmentation strategies 66, 68
    and comorbidity 66
    Combined SRI regimens 67
    SRIs and antipsychotics 66
    SRIs and behavior therapy 70
Aversion relief 25, 30

B

Basal ganglia 10, 11, 53, 54, 54–55,
   55, 56, 57, 58, 59, 68
Beck, Aaron *See* Beck's cognitive therapy
Beck's cognitive therapy 33, 35–36
    Efficacy 37
    Probability estimation 36
    Responsibility pie 36
Behavioral avoidance tests (BAT) 14, 15
Behavior assessment 14–15 *See*
   also Behavioral avoidance
   tests (BAT); SUDS
Behavior Therapy 4
Behavior therapy 13, 21, 23–31, 36, 39,
   40, 42, 43, 45, 46, 48, 57, 58, 70–71
    Early treatment methods 24–26
    Efficacy 29–31
    Exposure and response prevention
      26–29 *See also* Imagined exposure;
      In-vivo exposure; Response prevetion
    Resistance to 4
Biological treatments 30, 68–69
    Deep Brain Stimulation (DBS) 69
    Electroconvulsive Therapy (ECT) 69
    Neurosurgery 68–69 *See*
      also Cingulotomy; Capsulotomy
    Transcranial Magnetic
     Stimulation (TMS) 69
Bipolar disorder 53
Body dysmorphic disorder 8, 11, 15, 16–17
BuSpar® *See* Buspirone
Buspirone (BuSpar®) 66, 67

C

Capsulotomy 68
Caudate nucleus 53, 57, 58
Celexa® *See* Citalopram
Characteristics 1, 2, 7, 9,
   74 *See also* symptoms

Avoidance 9, 10, 13, 14, 15, 22,
   23, 30, 32, 39, 53, 74, 75
  Overestimating harm 9, 13, 33
  Overestimating importance of thoughts 9
  Worrying 1, 8, 9, 18
Checking 2
  and assessment 8, 13, 15,
   16, 17, 18, 19, 73, 74
  and pharmacotherapy 52, 71
  and psychotherapy 26, 29, 44, 45
Cingulotomy 68
Citalopram (Celexa®) 63
Cleaning 2
  and assessment 7, 74
  and pharmacotherapy 52, 71
  and psychotherapy 24, 26, 29, 44, 45
Clinical interviews 10–13, 14, 75
Clomipramine (Anafranil®) 61,
  62, 64, 65, 67, 68, 71
  Special concerns 61, 63
Clonazepam (Klonopin®) 66, 67, 68
Cognitive-behavioral therapy 13, 33, 45, 48, 71
Cognitive therapy 31, 32–37 *See*
  also individual therapies
  and intrusive experiences/ideas 32, 33, 35
  and irrational/erroneous beliefs 32, 33
  and negative automatic thoughts 35
  Beck's cognitive therapy 33, 35–36
  Efficacy 36–37
  Rational emotive therapy (RET) 34–35
Comorbidity 52, 53, 66
Compulsions 1
  and assessment 7, 8, 9, 10, 12, 13,
   14, 15, 16, 17, 18, 19, 74, 75, 76
  and pharmacotherapy 52, 71
  and psychotherapy 23, 24, 25, 26, 28,
   30, 31, 33, 34, 37, 38, 42, 45, 46
Compulsive Activity Checklist (CAC) 13
Contamination
  and assessment 9, 18, 73, 74, 75
  and pharmacotherapy 52
  and psychotherapy 23, 29, 36
Cyclic antidepressants 67
  Mirtazapine (Remeron®) 63, 67, 68
  Trazodone (Desyrel®) 67
  Venlafaxine (Effexor®) 67, 68

D

Deep Brain Stimulation (DBS) 69
Delusional disorder 11, 15, 17

Depression 11, 18, 35, 37, 43, 45, 53, 59, 63,
  66, 69 *See also* Major depressive disorder
Desyrel® *See* Trazodone
Diagnosis 7–19, 43, 57
  Assessment tools 10–15 *See*
   also individual tools
   Behavior assessment 14–15
    See also Behavioral avoid-
    ance tests (BAT); SUDS
   Clinical interviews 10–13, 14, 75
   Laboratory/physical exam
    findings 10, 15
   Psychometric assessments 10, 15, 73
   Self-report instruments 10,
    13–14, 73–74
   Structured interviews 10,
    13–14, 73, 75–76
  Children/adolescents 2, 11, 15, 76
  Differential 7, 15–19 *See*
   also individual disorders
  DSM-IV (TR) Criteria 8, 13, 75
DSM-IV (TR) Criteria 8, 13, 75

E

Effectiveness
  Medications vs. behavior therapy 70–71
  of medications 62, 63, 64–65, 67 *See*
   also individual medications
  of non-pharmaceutical biological
   treatments 68–69 *See*
   also individual treatments
  of psychotherapy 29–31 *See*
   also individual therapies
Effexor® *See* Venlafaxine
Electroconvulsive Therapy (ECT) 69
Ellis, Albert *See* Rational
  emotive therapy (RET)
Environmental influences 4, 21, 22, 51
Eskalith *See* Lithium
Ethnic minorities 3
Etiology 21, 47
  Environmental factors 4, 21, 22, 51
  Genetic factors 11, 12, 51, 51–53, 60
  Neurobiological factors 51, 53,
   59 *See also* individual brain
   structures, Neurotransmitters
Exposure and response prevention 24, 26,
  26–29, 30–31, 36, 37, 42, 43, 44, 45, 47, 48,
  68, 70, 70–71 *See also* Imagined exposure;
  In-vivo exposure, Response prevention

F

Family therapy 46–48
    Efficacy 48
    Treatment methods 46–47
Fluoxetine (Prozac®) 61, 62, 63, 64, 65
Fluvoxamine (Luvox®) 61, 62, 63, 64, 65
Functional impairment 3, 12

G

Gender 2, 3
Generalized anxiety disorder
    (GAD) 11, 15, 17, 53
Genetics 11, 12, 51, 51–53, 60 *See*
    also Etiology: Genetic factors
Group therapy 39–45, 46
    Efficacy 45
    Therapeutic factors 39–40
    Treatment methods 40–45

H

Haldol® *See* Haloperidol
Haloperidol (Haldol®) 66
Hoarding 2
    and assessment 18, 73, 74, 75
    and pharmacotherapy 52, 71
    and psychotherapy 30
Hypochondriasis 8, 11, 15, 17–18

I

Imagined exposure 24, 26, 27, 28, 30, 40, 45
Imagined flooding 25 *See also* Behavior
    therapy: Early treatment methods
Impulses 1, 8, 10, 18, 74
In-vivo exposure 24, 26, 26–27, 30, 40, 42, 44

K

Klonopin® *See* Clonazepam

L

Laboratory/physical exam findings 10, 15
Lithium (Eskalith®) 66
Luvox® *See* Fluvoxamine

M

Major depressive disorder 8, 15,
    18 *See also* Depression
MAOIs (Monoamine oxidase inhibitors) 67
    Phenelzine (Nardil®) 67

Tranylcypromine (Parnate®) 67
Marital disruption 3, 46
Medical history 10, 10–11, 16
Medication
    Antianxiety agents
        Buspirone (BuSpar®) 66, 67
        Clonazepam (Klonopin®) 66, 67, 68
        Oxazepam (Serax®) 67
    Antidepressants 57, 59, 61, 63,
        67, 68, 70 *See also* SRIs
        Cyclic antidepressants 67
        Mirtazapine (Rem-
            eron®) 63, 67, 68
        Trazodone (Desyrel®) 67
        Venlafaxine (Effexor®) 67, 68
        MAOIs (Monoamine oxi-
            dase inhibitors) 67
        Phenelzine (Nardil®) 67
    Antimanic agent
        Lithium (Eskalith®) 66
    Antipsychotics
        Haloperidol (Haldol®) 66
        Pimozide (Orap®) 66
    Atypical antipsychotics 66
        Olanzapine (Zyprexa®) 66
        Quetiapine (Seroquel®) 66
        Risperidone (Risperdal®) 66, 68
    Clomipramine (Anafranil®) 61,
        62, 64, 65, 67, 68, 71
        Special concerns 61, 63
    Effectiveness
        of non-SRI medications 67
        of other biological treatments 68–69
        of SRI medications 62, 63, 64–65
        vs. behavior therapy 70–71
    Side effects 19, 42, 61, 62, 63, 65, 67, 70
    SRIs (Serotonin reuptake inhibitors)
        See Clomipramine; SSRIs
    SSRIs (Selective serotonin reuptake
        inhibitors) 61, 62, 63, 64, 65, 67, 68
        Citalopram (Celexa®) 63
        Fluoxetine (Prozac®) 61,
            62, 63, 64, 65
        Fluvoxamine (Luvox®) 61,
            62, 63, 64, 65
        Paroxetine (Paxil®) 61,
            62, 63, 64, 65, 70
        Sertraline (Zoloft®) 61, 62, 63, 64, 65
Medications vs. behavior therapy 70–71
Medication treatment *See also* Medication
    Augmentation strategies 66, 68
    and comorbidity 66
    Combined SRI regimens 67

SRIs and antipsychotics 66
SRIs and behavior therapy 70
Treatment resistant (to
    medications) 65, 69
Mirtazapine (Remeron®) 63, 67, 68
Modeling 27 *See also* In-vivo exposure

N

Nardil® *See* Phenelzine
Neurobiological factors 51, 53,
    59 *See also* individual brain
    structures, Neurotransmitters
Neuroimaging studies 54, 55, 56–59
Neurosurgery 68 *See*
    also Cingulotomy; Capsulotomy
Neurotransmitters 21, 22, 54, 59, 60, 63, 69

O

Obsessions 1, 2
    and assessment 7, 8, 9, 12, 13,
        17, 18, 19, 74, 75, 76
    and pharmacotherapy 52, 67, 71
    and psychotherapy 22, 23, 24, 25, 26, 29,
        30, 32, 33, 34, 35, 37, 38, 42, 44, 45, 46
Obsessive Compulsive Inventory-
    Short Version (OCI-SV) 13, 73
Obsessive compulsive personality
    disorder 16, 18
Obsessive cues/rituals 10, 13, 24, 26
OCD due to a general medical condition 10
Olanzapine (Zyprexa®) 66
Orap® *See* Pimozide
Orbito-frontal brain regions 55, 58, 59
Ordering 2
    and assessment 8, 15, 73
    and pharmacotherapy 52
    and psychotherapy 29
Oxazepam (Serax®) 67

P

Padua Inventory (PI) 13, 73, 73–74
PANDAS (pediatric autoimmune
    neuropsychiatric disorders associated
    with streptococcal infections) 11, 55, 56
Panic disorder 11, 15, 17, 53
Paradoxical intention 24, 29,
    30 *See also* Behavior therapy:
    Early treatment methods
Parnate® *See* Tranylcypromine
Paroxetine 63

Paroxetine (Paxil®) 61, 62, 64, 65, 70
Patient insight 10, 13
Paxil® *See* Paroxetine
Phenelzine (Nardil®) 67
Phobias 14, 16, 18–19
Pimozide (Orap®) 66
Post-traumatic stress disorder 11, 15, 17
Pre-frontal brain region 55, 58
Prevalence 41
Prognosis 4, 10, 11, 12, 13
Prozac® *See* Fluoxetine
Psychiatric history 10, 11–12
Psychoanalytic therapy 23, 37–39
    Efficacy 39
    Treatment methods 38–39
Psychometric assessments 10, 15, 73
Psychotherapy 22, 39, 70, 71 *See*
    also individual therapies
    Behavior therapy 13, 21, 23–31, 36, 39,
        40, 42, 43, 45, 46, 48, 57, 58, 70–71
    Cognitive-behavioral therapy
        13, 33, 45, 48, 71
    Cognitive therapy 31, 32–37
    Effectiveness 29–31, 36–37, 39, 45, 48
    Family therapy 46–48
    Group therapy 39–45, 46
    Psychoanalytic therapy 23, 37–39
Psychotic disorder not otherwise
    specified 15, 17

Q

Quetiapine (Seroquel®) 66

R

Rational emotive therapy (RET) 33, 34–35, 37
    Effectiveness 37
    Ellis' ABC framework 34–35
Recovery rates 4
Remeron® *See* Mirtazapine
Repetitive checking behaviors 16, 19
Response prevention 24, 26, 26–29, 36,
    37, 40, 42, 43, 44, 45, 47, 48, 68, 70, 71
Risperdal® *See* Risperidone
Risperidone (Risperdal®) 66, 68
Rituals 2, 3
    and assessment 7, 10, 13, 15, 17, 18, 19, 75
    and pharmacotherapy 54, 58
    and psychotherapy 22, 23, 24, 25, 26, 28,
        29, 30, 31, 33, 34, 37, 38, 44, 46, 47
Role of relatives 10, 12–13, 46

S

Satiation 25, 29, 30 *See also* Behavior therapy: Early treatment methods
Schizophrenia 2, 11, 16, 19, 43, 60, 66
Schizotypal personality disorder 11, 66
Self-report instruments 10, 13–14, 73–74
    Compulsive Activity Checklist (CAC) 13
    Obsessive Compulsive Inventory-Short Version (OCI-SV) 13, 73
    Padua Inventory (PI) 13, 73, 73–74
    Vancouver Obsessional Compulsive Inventory (VOCI) 13, 73, 74
    Yale-Brown Obsessive Compulsive Checklist and Scale (Y-BOCS) 13
    Yale-Brown Obsessive Compulsive Checklist and Scale (Y-BOCS) — Self-Report Version 43, 73, 75–76
Serax® *See* Oxazepam
Seroquel® *See* Quetiapine
Serotonin hypothesis 22, 42, 59
Serotonin neurotransmission 22, 59, 60
    and SRI medications 59
    Physiology 60
Sertraline (Zoloft®) 61, 62, 63, 64, 65
Severity 3, 4
    and assessment 11, 12, 13, 76
    and psychotherapy 31, 43, 45
Sexual/religious obsessions 1
    and assessment 8, 16, 75
    and psychotherapy 30
Side effects 19, 42, 61, 62, 63, 65, 67, 70
Significant stressor(s) 11, 12
Social/occupational functioning 4, 8, 10, 12
Social/psychological influences
    See Environmental influences
SRIs (Serotonin reuptake inhibitors)
    See Clomipramine; SSRIs
SSRIs (Selective serotonin reuptake inhibitors) 61, 62, 63, 64, 65, 68
    Citalopram (Celexa®) 63
    Fluoxetine (Prozac®) 61, 62, 63, 64, 65
    Fluvoxamine (Luvox®) 61, 62, 63, 64, 65
    Paroxetine (Paxil®) 61, 62, 63, 64, 65, 70
    Sertraline (Zoloft®) 61, 62, 63, 64
Structured Clinical Interview for DSM-IV (SCID) 14, 75
Structured interviews 10, 13–14, 73, 75–76
    Anxiety Disorders Interview Schedule (ADIS) 14
    Structured Clinical Interview for DSM-IV (SCID) 14, 75

Yale-Brown Obsessive Compulsive Scale and Symptom Checklist — Interview version (Y-BOCS) 14, 43, 75, 75–76
Substance-induced anxiety disorder 16, 19
SUDS (Subjective Units of Distress scale) 14, 42, 43
Suicide 4, 35
Superstitions 7, 16, 19
Sydenham's chorea 10, 55, 56
Symmetry
    and assessment 75
    and pharmacotherapy 52, 67, 71
    and psychotherapy 29
Symptoms
    Anxiety 1
        and assessment 8, 16, 17, 18, 19
        and pharmacotherapy 53, 58, 59, 62, 66, 67
        and psychotherapy 22, 23, 24, 26, 27, 28, 29, 31, 32, 33, 34, 37, 38, 39, 42, 43, 46
    Checking 2
        and assessment 8, 13, 15, 16, 17, 18, 19, 73, 74
        and pharmacotherapy 52, 71
        and psychotherapy 26, 29, 44, 45, 47
    Cleaning 2
        and assessment 7, 74
        and pharmacotherapy 52, 71
        and psychotherapy 24, 26, 29, 44, 45
    Compulsions 1
        and assessment 7, 8, 9, 10, 12, 13, 14, 15, 16, 17, 18, 19, 74, 75, 76
        and pharmacotherapy 52, 71
        and psychotherapy 23, 24, 25, 26, 28, 30, 31, 33, 34, 37, 38, 42, 45, 46
    Contamination
        and assessment 9, 18, 73, 74, 75
        and pharmacotherapy 52
        and psychotherapy 23, 29, 36
    Fluctuation 4
    Hoarding 2
        and assessment 18, 73, 74, 75
        and pharmacotherapy 52, 71
        and psychotherapy 30
    Obsessions 1, 2
        and assessment 7, 8, 9, 12, 13, 17, 18, 19, 74, 75, 76
        and pharmacotherapy 52, 67, 71
        and psychotherapy 22, 23, 24, 25, 26, 29, 30, 32, 33, 34, 35, 37, 38, 42, 44, 45, 46
    Ordering 2

and assessment 8, 15, 73
and pharmacotherapy 52
and psychotherapy 29
Pervasiveness 12
Rituals 2, 3
    and assessment 7, 10, 13,
        15, 17, 18, 19, 75
    and pharmacotherapy 54, 58
    and psychotherapy 22, 23,
        24, 25, 26, 28, 29, 30, 31,
        33, 34, 37, 38, 44, 46, 47
Severity 3
    and assessment 11, 12, 13, 76
    and psychotherapy 31, 43, 45
Sexual/religious obsessions 1
    and assessment 8, 16, 75
    and psychotherapy 30
Symmetry
    and assessment 75
    and pharmacotherapy 52, 67, 71
    and psychotherapy 29
Symptom fluctuation 4
Symptom pervasiveness 12
Systematic desensitization 24, 28,
    29, 30 *See also* Behavior therapy:
    Early treatment methods

T

Thought stopping 25, 30 *See also* Behavior
    therapy: Early treatment methods
Tics 12, 16, 19, 53, 54, 56, 66 *See
    also* Tourette's syndrome
Tourette's syndrome 16, 19, 52, 53, 54, 66

Tourette's syndrome 12 *See also* Tics
Transcranial Magnetic Stimulation (TMS) 69
Tranylcypromine (Parnate®) 67
Trazodone (Desyrel®) 67
Treatment *See* Biological treatments;
    Medication; Psychotherapy
Treatment plan 11
Treatment resistant (to medications) 65, 69

V

Vancouver Obsessional Compulsive
    Inventory (VOCI) 13, 73, 74
Venlafaxine (Effexor®) 67, 68

Y

Yale-Brown Obsessive Compulsive
    Checklist and Scale (Y-BOCS) — Self-
    Report Version 13, 43, 73, 75–76
Yale-Brown Obsessive Compulsive Scale
    and Symptom Checklist — Interview
    version (Y-BOCS) 14, 43, 75, 75–76

Z

Zoloft® *See* Sertraline
Zyprexa® *See* Olanzapine

We Want Your Opinion!

Comments about **Obsessive Compulsive Disorder**:

_____

_____

_____

_____

_____

Other titles you would like Compact Clinicals to offer:

_____

_____

_____

_____

To be placed on our mailing list, please provide the following:

Name: _____

Address: _____

_____

_____

E-mail: _____

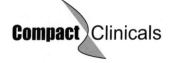

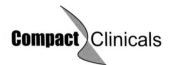

Order in 3 easy steps:

▶ 1   Provide complete billing and shipping information

Name_____   Company_____

Profession_____   Dept./Mail Stop_____

Street Address/P.O. Box_____

City/State/Zip_____

Telephone_____   ☐ Ship to Residence   ☐ Ship to Business

▶ 2   Choose Titles

For Clinicians:	Qty.	Unit Price	Total
Attention Deficit Hyperactivity Disorder *The latest assessment and treatment strategies*		$16.95	
Bipolar Disorder *The latest assessment and treatment strategies*		$16.95	
Borderline Personality Disorder *The latest assessment and treatment strategies*		$16.95	
Conduct Disorders *The latest assessment and treatment strategies*		$16.95	
Depression in Adults *The latest assessment and treatment strategies*		$16.95	
Obsessive Compulsive Disorder *The latest assessment and treatment strategies*		$16.95	
Post-Traumatic and Acute Stress Disorders *The latest assessment and treatment strategies*		$16.95	

For Physicians:

	Qty.	Unit Price	Total
Bipolar Disorder: Treatment and Management		$18.95	

	Subtotal
Continuing Education credits available for mental health professionals. *Call 1-800-408-8830 for details.*	**Tax** (Add 7.975% in MO)
	Shipping ($3.75 first book/ $1.00 per additional book)
	TOTAL

▶ 3   Choose Payment Method

Please charge my: ☐ Visa ☐ MasterCard ☐ Discover ☐ American Express   ☐ Check Enclosed

Account # __ __ __ — __ __ __ — __ __ __ __ — __ __ __ __   Exp. Date __ __ / __ __

Name on Card_____   Cardholder Signature_____

Postal Orders: Compact Clinicals, 7205 NW Waukomis Dr., Suite A, Kansas City, MO 64151

Telephone Orders: Toll Free 1-800-408-8830   **Fax Orders:** 1 (816) 587-7198